Still Crying
for Help

Sadia Messaili

Still Crying for Help

The Failure of
Our Mental Healthcare Services

Translated from the French by Aleshia Jensen

Baraka
Books

Montréal

Original title : *Les fous crient toujours au secours*
@ 2019, Les Éditions Écosociété. All rights reserved
Translation © Aleshia Jensen

ISBN 978-1-77186-227-1 pbk; 978-1-77186-231-8 epub; 978-1-77186-232-5 pdf

Cover design by Maison 1608
Book Design by Folio Infographie
Proofreading by Blossom Thom, Robin Philpot

Legal Deposit, 3rd quarter 2020
Bibliothèque et Archives nationales du Québec
Library and Archives Canada

Published by Baraka Books of Montreal

Printed and bound in Quebec

Trade Distribution & Returns
Canada – UTP Distribution: UTPdistribution.com

United States
Independent Publishers Group: IPGbook.com

We acknowledge the support, including translation support, from the Société de développement des entreprises culturelles (SODEC) and the Government of Quebec tax credit for book publishing administered by SODEC.

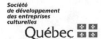

Société
de développement
des entreprises
culturelles
Québec

Funded by the Government of Canada
Financé par le gouvernement du Canada   Canadä

Contents

Foreword

A Story of Therapeutic Failure

When the loved ones of a person struggling with a mental health issue hear the words "psychosis" and "schizophrenia," their world falls apart. Some say they'd rather it have been cancer. It's this painful experience—the story of failed treatment rooted in today's reality—that Sadia Messaili recounts in *Still Crying for Help*, which in French is entitled *Les fous crient toujours au secours*. This title echoes the 1961 book by Jean-Charles Pagé *Les fous crient au secours*.[1] Diagnosed with schizophrenia, Sadia's son Ferid Ferkovic took his own life after being released from a second hospitalization. His journey through the mental health system unfortunately mirrors what many men and women have experienced after a first psychotic episode or a particularly intense depressive episode: they felt that they had no voice.

When someone has a psychotic episode, they are ultimately labelled irresponsible and are considered incapable of making decisions or possessing a reasonable opinion. They are not listened to, nor must they be. They are delusional. They believe that there is a mission they must complete or that the whole world is out to get them. And if this person expresses the wish not to be medicated and asks for alternative treatment, just as Ferid did, it's taken for granted they have no idea what they are saying. Those who we call the "mentally ill," particularly when in the throes of a psychotic episode, are stripped of humanity's most important attribute: reason. They are in some ways positioned out of this world, in a parallel universe, unattainable. Listening to them, entering into their delusions, means confirming this fantasy world is real. They must instead be brought back to reality.

When the staff imposed medical treatment on Ferid against his wishes, they erected a wall between them. How can you establish a therapeutic relationship under these conditions? How is it surprising that the staff lost his cooperation? Neuroleptics, also known as "antipsychotics," are major tranquilizers, powerful molecules that often inhibit motivation and the ability to think clearly and, consequently, one's ability to participate in one's own recovery. What Ferid was asking—to be treated in some way other than by drugs—was not the moon. Norway currently has psychiatric clinics and hospitals with unmedicated wards and beds where people can receive care in other forms.

Ferid came to the hospital the first time of his own free will, like many people in distress who know they need help. He would be treated with neuroleptics. Because they didn't work for him, the staff advised a more aggressive approach: electroshock treatment, which his mother would refuse. During his second hospitalization three years later, Ferid would refuse all medication, as was his right, and would attempt in vain to be heard.

For medical professionals trained in the arcane intricacies of biological psychiatry, turning to neuroleptics is a mandatory route. It's often the first and last option.

Current protocols in biopsychiatry maintain that schizophrenia is incurable and that patients must be medicated for the rest of their lives. When someone does manage to recover, they're told that likely it wasn't schizophrenia in the first place. Yet defining the illness as one that has clear and distinct boundaries, moving toward inevitable deterioration with no hope of healing, is being increasingly called into question. What we call "schizophrenia," as a unique entity, covers very different realities, and many psychiatrists propose replacing the term with the concept of a "spectrum of psychosis." When people are told they have an incurable condition, that they have no future, that their life will be full of suffering, do we not risk sending the message that perhaps they are "right" in wanting a way out?

Numerous experiments done on the selective use of neuroleptics, dating back to the early 1970s, note alternatives to the current paradigm. Here I will cite a few of the most recent. A long-term (20-year) study by Harrow and Jobe and a clinical trial by Wunderink (7 years) show that the people who best make it through their illness either discontinue medication or reduce the dose. While coming off drugs, which must be done very gradually and under the supervision of a mental health professional,[2] a person can relapse in the two to four years that follow, but discontinuing medication or reducing the dose can improve long-term results.

The Open Dialogue therapy developed in Finland's Lapland region has begun to extend its reach beyond the country's borders. The therapy advocates for minimal use of neuroleptics. Most of the people (67 percent) treated with this method after their first psychotic episode—including close follow-up, a multidisciplinary team, home visits and a mobilized support network—have not ever taken pills and, after five years of support, they go on to live normal lives. Only 17 percent of participants in the study needed to use medication for a prolonged period.[3] Today in Lapland the rate of schizophrenia has substantially decreased.[4] Another approach called "388" in Quebec involves a kind of therapy with minimal use of drugs and has been able to substantially reduce hospitalizations.

People have been able to quiet their voices without medication by participating in the Hearing Voices groups. This method was developed by Dutch psychiatrists Marius Romme and Sandra Escher. While the biopsychiatric approach aims to eradicate the voices with medication, since they are a symptom of the illness, Romme suggests we enter into dialogue with them, confront and answer them. Through training, the voices can be calmed, quieted and, in some cases, even utilized. Sera Davidov, from Hearing Voices in the Unites States, summarizes the movement's guiding principles: not assuming that psychosis is an illness and not prohibiting the person from believing this; allowing patients to interpret their own experiences; accepting that the voices are real without prejudice as to the cause of these experiences; accepting that the goal is not necessarily to get rid of the voices, it's up to the individual; and understanding that hearing voices isn't always a negative experience, even though for certain people it can be.[5]

While in certain cases medication can prove useful in the short term, in the long term it is for the most part ineffective and dangerous, as demonstrated by numerous studies. Here is an excerpt from the Toulouse university hospital centre's pharmacology newsletter. The April 2017 issue summarizes the conclusions of Catalan specialist Dr. Joan-Ramon Laporte's research findings:

In the treatment of schizophrenia and other types of psychoses, neuroleptics can improve "positive" symptoms, but have no effect or unfavourable effects on the "negative" symptoms.[6] The percentages of treatment failure (due to ineffectiveness or side effects that oblige treatment discontinuation) are from 60 to 80 percent over 6 to 18 months. [...] Continued and prolonged exposure to neuroleptics produces cerebral atrophy and an irreversible diminishment of cognitive function. The incidence and severity of extrapyramidal and metabolic effects increase with the length of treatment. Despite this, drug manufacturers and numerous clinical practice guides recommend treating psychotic patients for an indefinite amount of time. [...] Neuroleptics affect the extrapyramidal system, glucose metabolism, vascular regulation and sexual function, among other things. They increase the mortality rate (5 to 6 percent, compared to 2 to 3 percent under placebo) through various mechanisms, particularly pneumonia, ventricular arrhythmias, stroke and femoral fractures. In one of the clinical trials spanning 18 months, the incidence of moderate or severe side effects was 67 percent (mainly excessive sedation, anticholinergic effects, extrapyramidal effects and sexual dysfunction). Generally the neuroleptics that most often produce extrapyramidal effects are the least likely to produce metabolic effects.[7]

In short, medication can be useful during the acute phase and can sometimes relieve symptoms in the short term for a certain percentage of people, but at a price: the drugs often trigger side effects that are worse than the symptoms being treated. Over 18 months, they fail in up to 80 percent of cases and are accompanied by a long list of terrifying side effects. Life expectancy for people diagnosed with schizophrenia is 15 to 20 years less than average life expectancy.

Biopsychiatry considers psychological distress and behaviour problems to be diseases of the brain, mainly if not entirely determined by genetics. This medical paradigm has been passed down to us from Emil Kraepelin (1856–1926), a Swiss-German doctor practicing around the turn of the last century who is recognized as one of the fathers of modern psychiatry. The view is based on the concordance rate among identical and fraternal twins (when one of the twins presents a given trait, the other presents the same trait). When concordance rates are higher in identical twins compared to fraternal twins, we attribute this to a genetic difference.

For schizophrenia, the American Psychiatric Association's *Diagnostic and Statistical Manual* of Mental Disorders claims that the rate is around 50 percent in identical twins, much higher than the rate with fraternal twins. If the "spectrum of psychosis" was strictly based on genetics, we would need a concordance rate closer to 100 percent. The 50 percent rate is the average for studies carried out since 1928. Yet the latest, most rigorous of these studies show much lower concordance rates of around 23 percent. In addition, to attribute these concordance rate differences to genetic factors, one would have to put forward the hypothesis that identical and fraternal twins experience environments that are largely equivalent. Yet, the "equal environment assumption" for identical and fraternal twins has been disproven.[8]

Since the human genome was sequenced in 2003 and epigenetics (the way the environment modifies gene expression) was developed, the old model brandished by genetic determinists—genes, proteins, traits, illnesses—has become obsolete. We have around 22,000 genes and, according to some estimates, between 100,000 and 250,000 (or up to a million) proteins.

After realizing that humans have so few genes (it was believed there were around 100,000), J. Craig Venter, a leader in research into genome sequencing, relegated genetic determinism to the past. With the exception of around 2 percent of the population which carry mutations in a handful of genes that can cause terrible and debilitating diseases, the strict deterministic vision, when it comes to explaining complex human traits and behaviour, is out of date.[9]

Epigenetics reveals that environments cause the same gene to act completely differently. It explains why a turtle's egg can hatch either male or female, depending on the incubation temperature, and a bee will become either the queen or a worker depending on the way it is fed.

Social, ecological and cultural factors are the biomedical model's blind spot—it assumes people live in a vacuum. To give two of many examples, young girls who have been sexually abused are 15 times more likely to develop a psychosis,[10] and black Caribbeans living in the United Kingdom are nine times more likely to develop a psychosis than the white UK population, while the rate of psychosis among black Caribbeans in their own country is not more elevated than that of the white UK population.[11]

Sadia's story and Ferid's journey show the failings of the system in handling mental distress (for the person concerned but also their loved ones) and the need for a more humane approach to care that takes patient's own wishes into account and provides adequate information and support for the people around them. This story highlights the importance of developing care that is more respectful of people. Those in need of help cannot be reduced to a set of symptoms or summed up with a diagnosis. They are a whole—a living, breathing person with a story. Care needs to take into account all of this. It is what could have helped, we would have hoped, to bring about a happier ending for Ferid and his family.

J.-Claude St-Onge

Our misfortune is not to be found in our fight with schizophrenia, but rather in the fight we had with people who decided to "treat" it their way.

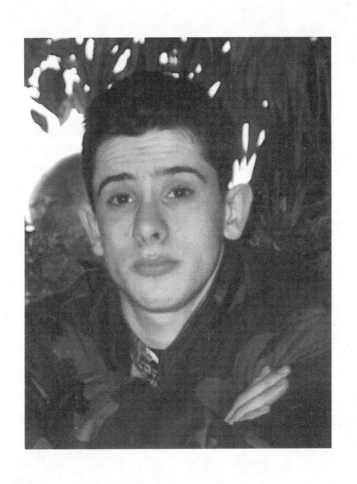

1. Deux-Montagnes, April 21, 2013

> "The way that we judge others and others judge us, we should hope to borrow their awareness and lend them ours."
> –Louis Joseph Mabire, *Dictionnaire de maximes* (1830)

I'd avoided leaving Montreal those last months. But on that cold Sunday in April 2013, sitting in the Saint-Eustache arena, I watch my four-year old grand-daughter Mila glide across the ice at her very first figure skating performance, so small among the other young skaters in her group. My mind is only half there, as I anxiously try to will time to speed up.

We don't make it back to Montreal until around five that evening. I go straight upstairs to look for my eldest son, Ferid. When I don't find him, I figure he's resting downstairs in his basement suite. I go back outside to check, but his front door is locked. My daughter Jasmina, Mila's mother, hasn't left yet. She flashes me a worried look and peers through the small window into his living room, then gives up. Maybe Ferid went for a walk, I think. Jasmina kisses me good-bye and heads home.

I go about things as usual, busying myself with supper for my two sons. But I can't focus. I go back outside as dusk is slowly setting in. If Ferid went to the store or for a walk, as he often does, he'd have been home long before now.

Outside I squeeze under the landing to get near his bedroom window. The room is empty, pitch black. The bed is still made. Leaning against the mattress is a bag with the pillow he took with him two days earlier to spend the night at Jasmina's in Deux-Montagnes. Ferid had agreed to go visit her, which was a first. We'd all had a nice, happy evening together. Early the next day, he'd wanted to go back to Montreal. His face had been pale and he was trembling all over. I told him I'd come with him, but he assured me it wasn't necessary. My daughter's partner, Pablo, had driven him back. I knew he needed to rest, to have some time to himself. It was a miracle he'd agreed to come with us in the first place.

I duck back out from under the landing. I can feel anxiety rise in my chest. My mind starts conjuring explanations, all sorts of scenarios. He's out. He'll be home soon. He walked to Sherbrooke Street to pick up a few things, as he often does. He's a grown man: sensible and cautious. I think back to the bag on the floor of his room: he hasn't used his pillow since he got back, that means. Maybe he slept upstairs? But it didn't look as though he had.

I go back down and knock on the door. There's no movement, no lights on inside. My heart races. I go back upstairs, grab the spare key for the door out back, and fly down the stairs. I slam my body against his kitchen door, but it doesn't budge. I pull on the handle in vain. Terrified and imagining the worst, I try to break down the damn door. I had never imagined it to be so solid. I go back upstairs and call Majid, Ferid's dad, and tell him that Ferid has locked himself in the basement, that he needs to get over here right away. Majid tells me not to panic, and I yell at him to hurry.

Thoughts assail me—terrible thoughts. I hold my head in my hands and beg Allah to save me. I pace my bedroom, trying to bargain with God. "Please, not this! Not this! Let me carry the burden, God. Anything but this!" Everything fades and all I can focus on is this overwhelming thought that has lodged itself in my mind.

Majid comes over with a friend. The two men try to get the door to Ferid's suite open, and it eventually gives way. Majid calls his son's name. He walks past the half-open bathroom door and cries out, "*Ferid, no...!*" My blood goes cold. I'm standing directly behind him. In a flash I catch sight of my son lying in the bathtub, his face serene and his eyes closed, asleep. His father kneels next to him, cradles Ferid's head in his arms and speaks to him in a soft plaintive voice. I can't bring myself to get any closer. Maybe he's still breathing, I think. Is he still breathing?—did

I say those words aloud? Did Majid gesture or say something to me, or did I see it in his eyes? I back out of the room, howling like an animal in the night. My cries rise and fill the dark apartment. I double over, struck by the unnameable violence of death. In an instant, my life splits in two.

Outside I sank to the ground on the main-floor landing and stared into the dark, deserted street. I laid there in total shock for I don't know how long. Then I got up and called 911. I have no memory of what I said. The dispatcher couldn't understand me, so Adam, my younger son, grabbed the receiver and told the person on the line someone was dead, that they should send the police right away. Had he already then taken on the role of protector? Taking care to bring me to the couch, stroking my face and stemming the flow of lamentations with his sweetness. He nestled close to me while his father waited in the basement for the police officers to arrive.

Everything came rushing to the surface like lava. The entirety of my son's suffering which I had watched as a powerless mother expanded in my chest. The struggles, the dashed hopes, the tremendous effort it had taken to live one hour at a time, the pain he'd pushed down to make himself as small as possible, as little of a burden as he could—all this flashed before me in overwhelming clarity. My eldest son is no longer there for me to take in my arms. I can no longer tell him how much I love him and that I'm here for him. I'd never be able to hold him in my arms again.

The police arrived first, then the paramedics, then the investigating officer. That irreversible action. The word we don't say aloud. The unimaginable. The thing we have to face, and its permanence. It was only the start of what would be a long night. I was angry at myself that I hadn't been home, that I'd let my guard down, that I hadn't done enough for Ferid. Adam cried and hugged me, telling me, "Ferid's not suffering anymore, Mom... He's not suffering anymore—it's all over," searching for solid ground to stand on so he could steady me too. The night was long and empty. I felt utterly alone.

Majid's partner, Sara, arrived at the house. It was thanks to her that I didn't end up completely dehydrated. I had cried out all the water in my body. In that moment, I thanked God for giving humans the gift of tears to heal our wounds. We turned on the computer and put on the Holy Quran. The recitation of the verses reminding Man of the need to accept his impermanence in order to reach an eternal afterlife free of suffering produced a spiritual effect that, at times, managed to calm me. Pain gradually took over my body, carving out a space inside me—a deep chasm that I'd carry with me for a long time.

The team in the basement cordoned off the area. Our child's body had to be taken away for a possible autopsy. Around two in the morning, we prepared to notify our loved ones. My first thought was to call my daughter, but I wanted to wait till morning. Instead I called my sister Amina; we were very close, and her support helped sustain me throughout. She stayed with me for hours on Skype then took charge of telling the rest of the family. Djamel, my younger brother who lived in Montreal, came to the house the next morning.

Ferid was my parents' first grandson. He was born on March 21, 1981 in Zagreb, his father's hometown and where Majid and I had met in November 1979. During a particularly difficult period in my life as a young mother, I'd made the difficult decision to send him to my parents in Algeria. Ferid was four. My relationship was on the rocks. I was expecting another child and working nights. Without any family support in Zagreb to help me look after my young son, whose father had given up his role as a parent, I was on my own.

I spoke to Ferid's pediatrician about what would be best for him under the circumstances. He helped me decide: a safe, loving environment for a set amount of time was the best possible option, in his opinion. Ferid didn't know his maternal grandparents and didn't speak a word of Arabic. It would just be for a few months, I thought, until I had the baby and could decide what to do next.

This separation was no doubt a first trauma for Ferid, one that he had a hard time recovering from. In addition to learning Arabic, then French—his mother tongue was Croatian—Ferid also had a mild stutter; though, as a child, it never proved a hindrance to his academic success or social life.

When his sister was born, in June 1985, his father and I reconciled and went back to Algeria to get Ferid. I'll never forget his reaction when we got there: he'd been waiting for us for such a long time, but when he saw his sister in my arms, he turned his back to me and refused to kiss me hello. The situation soon smoothed over, of course, and he and Jasmina became inseparable.

Everyone adored Ferid: my Croatian friend Vesna, my sisters—especially Amina. He was handsome, energetic, sweet and mischievous. He'd often go with my brother and his friends to the sea. We take the things we hold dear for granted, forgetting that they belong to God. In beautiful, plentiful, golden Algeria, tormented by political storms, planting roots is a heroic feat. But in some ways, we were happy there.

I'd come back to Algeria for various reasons, including Croatia's worsening economic situation, which preceded the brutal ethnic wars in the former Yugoslavia—wars that left approximately 150,000 dead, mainly Bosniaks. But civil war was also simmering in Algeria, conflict took root at the very heart of a people constantly caught in the political crossfire. Everyone was in the line of fire: intellectuals, dissidents, women and even children. And foreigners, a group we belonged to due to my marriage to a non-Algerian, were a visible minority and targets; different terrorist groups openly claimed responsibility for these attacks. So we prepared for exile, like so many other Algerian nationals.

We left the country on July 29, 1993. Ferid was 12 years old.

2. April 22, 2013:
The First Day Without Ferid

I try to recall the first day. Did I close my eyes for a single moment? Did I wait till dawn to say the first prayer of the day? Did I keep my wits about me enough to carry out, one by one and with love and respect, the tasks required to help my son reach his final resting place? How did I make it through the minefield of emotions as I prepared to mourn a loss I had so feared? The news of a child's death always made me think first of the devastated parents, and I barely dared to imagine the nightmare ahead of them. I'd prayed to God to put me to any test but this one. But fate, which some may call by another name, has its own logic. Any wavering in my faith up till that point, any skepticism that may have crept through the cracks, was counterbalanced by the abundance of compassion I received—it's what kept me on my feet. Like in times of great human catastrophe, every ounce of compassion, every gesture made, however small, is vital. It rallies us together.

That morning we finally call my son-in-law. We ask him to come as quickly as he can, and to bring Jasmina, without saying more. Then more phone calls. Our family and friends in France, England, Algeria, Croatia, and Morocco quickly learn the news, some from my siblings, others through social media. Everyone who knew him speaks to us about what a rich life he lived and how much he meant to them. Jasmina literally collapses when she hears the news. She is riddled with guilt since we were at her house, far from Ferid, when he breathed his final breath, alone. Could she have prevented something we couldn't have seen coming? "I should have insisted you go home with him, Mom..." These are the inevitable thoughts that would haunt us, the pain we'd be unable to chase.

But we would support each other and move through the grief hand in hand. Ferid had predicted as much. He'd often mentioned in his last days the importance of love. "Make a circle, Mom," he would say, interlacing his fingers. He repeated to me softly: "Stay united. Support each other. Stay connected." He knew our needs better than any of us. He brought us together.

My brother took charge of the funeral arrangements and communicating with the mosque. When a Muslim dies, the burial must take place within 24 hours, before sunset. Islamic funeral rites are of great importance. But my son's body would only be released three days later, on April 24. No autopsy had been performed. The official cause of death given was suicide by carbon monoxide, from the small container of burnt charcoal found in the bathroom. Accepting those terrible findings written on the coroner's report would be a difficult process—a loss of two kinds. What were Ferid's true intentions that night?

3. April 24, 2013: The Day of Departure

"Say: truly the death that you run away from, then it will be truly that which you encounter.
After that you will be returned
to the One who has knowledge
of the unseen and the visible.
Then He will tell you what you had been doing."
—*The Sublime Quran,* Chapter 62, The Congregation, Verse 8 (Translated by Laleh Bakhtiar)

Ferid's body is brought straight to the mosque for the funeral rites that will deliver his soul to rest. Islam honours the person, in life and in death. When a Muslim dies, the body is washed, scented and shrouded. We pray for departed, bury them and invoke Allah's name in their favour. Pablo volunteers to represent the family for this rite. The funeral prayer is a community obligation (*fard kifaya*), so if some of the individuals perform it, the rest of the community may be discharged of the duty.

We go to the mosque, alongside our relatives, friends and acquaintances. Everyone makes a silent prayer next to Ferid's body, prays for his soul, and offers us their condolences. One sentence unites us in common destiny and reminds us that we belong to God: *"Inna lillahi wa inna ilayhi raji'un"* (Truly! To Allah we belong and truly, to Him we shall return).

The imam takes my son's body for the funeral prayer, which must take place in a room reserved for men. Just then, a group of beautiful women in western attire step into the mosque with a giant bouquet of flowers. It's my Quebec colleagues, who insisted on attending the funeral. Everyone behaves admirably, treating them with respect and gratitude, and we offer them a place at our sides.

We pray together and accept the condolences of everyone in attendance. Then the procession, several cars long, drives to the cemetery. Wednesday, April 24, 2013: as sweet and peaceful as the day Ferid was born. I was spared the pain of having to stand with the men, as I buried my eldest son.

Simplicity, equality, serenity and communion. This is what you feel as you stand before all the graves, all identical, except for a smaller one here or there indicating where a young child has been buried.

4. Ferid: Before

My son was an energetic little boy like all the other kids his age, despite everything he had lived through in those early years. I'll never forget the long, gruelling hospitalization for celiac disease—a diagnosis that had been determined after much difficulty when he was just 18 months old; then all the uprooting, family separations, exile, and the loss of the familiar, of extended family and friends. We were unstable parents in constant turmoil, as much due to cultural differences and often-conflicting needs as to the ongoing upheaval in both our countries, which blew through our lives like high winds, forcing us to keep packing up and seeking refuge elsewhere.

As a child born in the aftermath of war myself, I'd always found happiness to be out of reach. I'd been uprooted from the heights of a Moroccan paradise—Casablanca, La blanche—and transplanted in haste to a hostile land, a tiny village in western Algeria where the poor, uneducated residents wanted nothing to do with us, the Berber, the Kabyle, and where being different stamped you with the seal of rejection. At this early age

I had already slipped into the grey haze of what we call depression, a kind of protective shell that kept others at a safe distance and shut out the tumult of the world. Growing up in a state of emergency, fleeing had become a defense mechanism. My life was a high-speed train hurtling forward, one that never stopped long at any station.

In 1986, Algeria was still relatively peaceful. We arrived without any real plan. I found work teaching and interpreting almost right away, but my husband waited many long months for a temporary permit that would allow him to work on a housing construction project for a Croatian company that had been awarded the contract. After several miserable months under my parents' roof, we pulled ourselves back to our feet. We were poor but obstinate, living in a beautiful country full of oil where, paradoxically, nothing ever belonged to the people. Social housing sprung up like mushrooms across the country, but remained inaccessible to the general population. Public funds used to build this housing for those in need—underprivileged people unable to think beyond their basic needs such as food and water, and shortages thereof—became business opportunities for the already well-positioned mafia. It was an open secret. Say you woke up one morning determined to get one of these so-called social lodgings. First, you'd have to find the source, generously grease the palm of someone who, thanks to a corrupt system, lets you live there without providing any official documents proving your right to do so. It was essentially the purchase and rental of public property to the state, through the same corrupt channels. And you could forget about filing a complaint. To whom, exactly, would you complain?

Getting a job involved the same wheeling and dealing. Without the right leads, unless you'd managed to get a government job or owned your own business, for most highly educated Algerians navigating the job market meant walking a tight-rope that might go slack at any moment. Family was the only safety net. Family or gold. Algerian immigrants packed up to find somewhere better, away from the danger, injustice, corruption, violence and the fear of being persecuted for their beliefs. When they were willing, women were offered the "privilege" of bartering sought-after advantages in exchange for their virtue. Many fell prey, due to a lack of education, resources and social justice.

All of us lived as a family in the Oran region until 1988, the same year Ferid would endure a second separation. My husband and I returned to Zagreb, leaving the children with my relatives. I told myself that my parents, five sisters, and three brothers would be there for them, would love and protect them. But it's impossible to know what goes on in the mind of a child, when nothing has really been explained to them. After six months, exhausted by grief, I returned to Algeria alone, leaving their father in Croatia to settle his work problems. Often unawareness, optimism, obligation and ignorance translate into a sense of resilience. But these separations deeply affected me.

As social ills multiplied, the Algerian people rose up at the start of the 1990s, demanding a multi-party system and other political change. But at a high price. Algeria would enter a down-ward spiral in the 1990s, leading to ten years of civil war. In this complex climate, numer-ous guerilla movements went underground to overthrow the regime and establish an Islamic state. Officials, teachers, journalists, intellec-tuals and artists were targeted and murdered under the pretext of being government support-ers. Foreigners were ordered to leave the country, or risk being killed.

My family, especially my father, shielded us. I soon found myself out of work, discriminated against for being married to a foreigner. But I didn't give up. I found another job with an oil company, which paid for a roof over our heads; in other words, a trailer with one bedroom, a liv-ing room, kitchen and bathroom. It was one of the makeshift shelters American companies had abandoned once their contracts with the local oil company expired. They've since been fixed up and serve as mansions for the many families who came to the Arzew district seeking work.

By the time Majid came back to Algeria, the social climate was even stormier. He loved

Algeria, but his status as a foreigner had become a problem. There was no question of him living there, even temporarily, let alone working. At the police station where I went to plead his case, the officers were evasive, even hostile. I was told: "Stay on as a tourist. Don't ask for anything." Though foreigners were caught in the crossfire of terrorist groups and criminals, Algerians— most of them civilians—would be the main victims of the fratricides led in the name of political demands and almost completely disconnected from the will of the people.

That's when I promised myself that I'd never again be separated from my children. Whatever happened, we'd stay together. So Majid and I got back on the road to exile with our two kids. How did Ferid and his sister experience yet another uprooting? What effect did it have, the permanent loss of dreams, friendships, love and sunshine we associated with the humble little dwelling where we left everything behind (and that was vandalized the moment we had gone)? My daughter Jasmina would sometimes recall moments laced with sadness or happy memories there. But not Ferid— other than bits and pieces about how fun it used to be playing with the kids in the tiny camp, where our family had spent a relatively stable eight years.

This was the journey in search of utopian peace. In my book *La route de la dignité*,[1] I tell the story of our crash landing into precarity and survival. Today, considering the fate of many 21st century refugees, it seems humanity has become dangerously acclimatized to terror. We first arrived in Austria, where we were safe but anonymous, in transit to an unknown host country. Ferid spent his early teens there, with a greatly impoverished social life. He was an easy-going child with a single school friend named Miralem, a gentle, caring young Bosnian boy.

Then in December 1995, we stepped onto Quebec soil for the first time. We had to adapt to the new country and climate, and throw our all into it. Ferid was 14. He'd become more reserved with age, much like myself. He was brilliant at math and dreamed of becoming a pilot one day. He was shy, but had friends who he spent much of his time with. In 1997, his brother Adam was born and two years later, the family was fractured for good when their father and I divorced. I became the sole earner and had to rely on the older two to look after their younger brother while I was at work. I figured we were mostly out of the woods.

Ferid began advanced math classes after scoring high on his Secondary 5 exams, so that he could apply to an air force training program. He scored 99 percent on his exams! That was *before*. Back when I thought everything would go smoothly. That all I had to do was persevere. I finished a bachelor's degree in inclusive education, which you needed to teach in Quebec, and began working two days a week at an elementary school in Ville Saint-Laurent.

My children were everything to me. I wanted the best for them. I made sure they finished high school, pushing for them to go as far in life as they could. I also dreamed of owning a house. Though I was still dependant on social assistance, which provoked both shame and humiliation in me, I wanted to buy a house. It was what we'd always lacked at each failed resettling and what signified security in my eyes.

In 2000, my parents came to Quebec as visitors. They stayed for a year. Ferid spent little time with them during their visit, but as everyone knows, teenagers prefer the company of friends. He went to La Ronde with his friends, had them over to the house, laughed and spent quality time with his little brother, Adam. The skies were still clear.

Ferid explained to me that applying for the air force program wasn't easy: the program required high math grades, but also a pristine bill of health. Every candidate file was carefully studied. The process generally took a year. His father and I discussed with Ferid the issues related to his choice of career: being a pilot in the air force could mean dropping bombs on people. No matter the reason or who was targeted, he would be trained to kill. We had this discussion only once. We wanted to respect his decision. Knowing the admission process wouldn't be easy, we hoped it would give him time to think about his choice.

In the meantime came the 9/11 terrorist attacks and their lasting impact. During that period, I also began teaching full time. Ferid checked in several times on his application's progress, but he found the admission criteria tough, especially in terms of physical endurance. Little by little he began to give up the idea, to our great relief. He seemed to lose interest in anything but the present.

Today, I wonder why I stayed at school those two extra hours each day to plan lessons and projects. I'd come home late, then deal with the family duties, which fell to me as head of a single-parent household. Time erodes our memories until there's almost nothing left. The fragments I've held onto are marked by the frenetic pace that life imposes when each hour is planned out. For an immigrant, the first years are crucial in finding a place in a host society, especially in the job market.

In September 2002, I began urging Ferid to apply to Cégep. With his grades, he'd have his pick of schools. He patiently explained that he had no idea what he wanted to study. I came up with suggestions: meet with a guidance counselor, visit colleges... I urged Ferid to keep his sights high, just as I'd been taught to do. I anticipated his successes. I kept my mind on the future, often to the detriment of the present. And eventually he gave in. He did what I asked and began venturing out of the house. And I could finally breathe easy. Or so I thought. At the end of the day, parents are parents. No one else lives through the same worries or guilt. When we do too much, we think we haven't done enough. And though we know our limits, we suffer from our inevitable powerlessness. To hide it, we do what we do best: push onward and force others to do the same.

In 2002, we finally move into a new house. It needs to be renovated, but I'm proud. I've finally been given a permanent position at work. I pay more attention to my daughter, who is full swing into her teens. I try to be present. My physical presence isn't enough, but I trust in our lucky stars and our incredible resilience. Adam only sees his father on weekends, and this absence hits him hard. Ferid spends more time in his tiny room, playing video games day and night.

5. Ignorance

I've always loved my son. With the kind of love that can sometimes start to smother, until the other person can't breathe. Love I expressed through expectations, pressure and other ways that drove Ferid to say or do things to escape its grasp. When I insisted he at least eat at the table with us, or that he do something other than just sleep and play video games, it was like speaking to a brick wall. So I sought out help and a place where I could talk. Since I couldn't convince Ferid to see a specialist, I went to parent support groups—associations that guide, listen, inform and assist.

My background, culture, values and beliefs meant that I encouraged my children to learn, become independent and plan for their future. Maybe Ferid had a health problem or was going through a temporary crisis; whatever the case, I needed to find a solution. What worried me most was the near complete breakdown in communication between Ferid and everyone else. We'd grown afraid of approaching him. Sometimes he'd slip quietly out of his room to eat something.

He'd stand at the counter, glaring at us with an unnerving distrust so unlike him if he happened to catch one of our worried looks.

The situation was painful and distressing, and we felt helpless. I sought professional help so I could better understand what Ferid might be going through. The answer was always the same, and for good reason: the young person has to seek help, not their parents. An educator at the nearby Tandem crisis centre on Rue Côte-Saint-Antoine explained that in the case of an adult, there's nothing the parents can do. My son had to ask for help of his own accord. The young man I spoke to was sympathetic nonetheless and took the time to reassure me. "It might be that your son just wants a break," he explained. "A lot of young people don't know what they want to do after high school. All the different options can sometimes be overwhelming. Maybe he'll decide to get a job and continue his studies later on."

The possibility of going back to school whenever you want was simply not a reality in the countries where I've lived. Elsewhere, it's a straight path from elementary to university, provided you get in. Going backwards isn't an option. This trajectory, inspired by the French model, means that time is not our own and can't be altered as we please. Here, it's not unusual for young people to take a break. I just had to be patient. But my anxiety started to well up, and I panicked. Once again, I turned to psychology. I can still hear one psychologist's voice as she painted a dark future ahead: a young man who'd turn inward to the point of no return. She had once again pelted me with the same words, her tone implying the obvious: parents can't be the ones to seek help, even if their concerns are well-founded.

Our family dynamics shift. We don't avoid Ferid, but we increasingly fear his reactions. He's still in touch with two or three friends, but they're always the ones to visit him. One day one of them tells me he's worried. He says he doesn't think Ferid is doing well, that the sooner we get him out of his room the better. Adam remarks that his big brother does nothing except play video games all day and says he wants to do the same when he grows up. Adam is five years old and looks up to his older brother.

One day, Ferid tells me he's had a horrible nightmare and odd sensations. I don't understand, but I listen and try to reassure him. I try to quell my panic as my guilt grows. I feel powerless. Ferid is 21 now. His father and I decide something needs to be done. We want him to learn how to stand on his own two feet and we ask him to move out. And get a job. We hope he'll slowly learn to look after a small apartment, take care of his own space and pay his own bills. It's immensely painful for me to force him out of the nest, but I brush these feelings aside for his own good. We reassure him that we'll support him no matter what: "We'll help you, Ferid. You won't be alone. We'll pay your rent until you find work. We just want you to have the opportunity to live well. And then you'll be able to make your own choices."

Ferid has never been very open or forthcoming with his feelings. When I look into his beautiful eyes I see a whole world of sadness. A sadness full of resignation. One that will remain a painful memory for me. I know I'm rushing him. It's difficult for me. And I feel a profound sense of guilt as a little voice whispers in my ear that this works out well for me, that I'm looking forward to getting him out of the house so I can rest and live my own life—it's a feeling that cuts deep. But I quickly fall into my supportive role; I go with him to apply for social assistance, and his dad finds him an apartment near his own. His father is quick to offer him a job doing renovation, but the work is difficult, unpleasant and poorly paid. The entire experience is painful for Ferid, and the failure weighs down my motherly suffering even more.

Six months later and things are looking up. Ferid seems happy. He visits from time to time. He's taking a training course and has been working for a while now as a security guard. He seems to have reconnected with a few friends. I don't hear from him often, but I'm hopeful again. I visit his apartment once or twice. It strikes me as clean and spacious, and I breathe a sigh of relief. On Mother's Day, Ferid comes over and we all go out to eat. His face is glowing.

Ferid moves to a new apartment. Little by little, the distance wedges a gap between us. He doesn't visit anymore. News is sporadic and usually it comes via his father, but I stay positive. Then Majid's marital problems begin complicating things with him and Ferid. Another wound. I fall back into a cycle of guilt and sadness. I make a few attempts to visit him, but he won't open the door.

A hellish loneliness stretched from 2005 to 2008, for both Ferid and me. I couldn't understand what was preventing my beautiful boy from carving out a life for himself in the world and finding happiness. Guilt had become a second skin. He'd move to a new apartment, and I'd track him down each time, just to be able to see his face. When I'd ring the bell, he'd lift the curtain and look through the glass, and I'd catch a glimpse of him. Pale, and sad. I'd stand there at the doorstep pleading with him. I'd leave crying and return home with a heavy heart.

I continued to seek out professional help. Depending on the details I related, the response was neither reassuring nor worrying. It could be depression, they said. We're okay with depression. Why wouldn't we be? Even babies suffer from it, it seems. Ferid stopped talking to everyone in the family except his father, who he'd once been very close to. It was the only link left with our family.

In early June 2008, I decide to recontact Tandem for help. The situation has escalated beyond worry. We fear the worst. The staff at Tandem tell me I might be able to force my son to undergo a psychiatric assessment. They explain the significance of what we are considering doing and the fairly traumatic procedures involved.

The Act respecting the protection of persons whose mental state presents a danger to themselves or to others[1] governs confinement in a psychiatric institution. It states that, in certain precise and exceptional circumstances, the hospital may be authorized to detain a person without their consent.

If a doctor considers the mental state of a person to present a serious danger to themselves or to others, the person can be kept in the hospital against their will for a maximum of 72 hours. This is called **preventive confinement**. There are no precise criteria to define the danger related to a mental state. The physician's opinion is often based on the testimony of third parties (police officers or family members) as well as talk with the person and observation of their behaviour.

Temporary confinement is used to keep a person past the maximum 72-hour period of preventive confinement and to have the person submit to a psychiatric assessment (involving two examinations) to determine if their mental state presents a danger to themselves or to others. Temporary confinement must be ordered by a judge from the Quebec Court, but the request can be made by a member of a crisis intervention unit or a family member. The maximum duration is 96 hours.

And finally, **authorized confinement** must be obtained by the hospital from the Quebec Court in order to keep the person longer. It is granted if a judge deems the mental state of the person to present a danger to themselves or to others; the judge determines the duration of this confinement.

On June 15, 2008, Majid and I fill out and submit forms to request a psychiatric assessment.[2] The next day I appear in court. I explain the situation to the judge, who grasps its urgency and immediately orders a psychiatric assessment. In other words, temporary confinement.

I leave the courtroom in tears and head straight to the local police station. Everything happens very quickly. It feels like a dream. A wave of emotion washes over me: sorrow, sadness, fear and relief. Three police cars pull out of the station, on their way to request that my son follow them to the hospital. The officers are young, hard-working, compassionate and kind, and know how to handle this kind of situation. They explain to me what will happen. And it's awful. They'll surround the house and then knock on the door and ask Ferid to go with them. They warn me that what's about to happen will be difficult to watch. Ferid will probably have to be handcuffed. They also warn me that he'll be angry at me and that I shouldn't try to approach him. Everything feels surreal. It's not me there listening, it's some other mother somewhere else. I'm on the verge of falling apart.

The police officers silently disperse to all sides of the building and check the exits—it's an experience I wish on no parent. My son comes out with his frail body bent over and his hands in cuffs, walking forward compliantly. I wring my hands and pray. I look for God inside myself and up in the perfectly clear sky.

I hope this will be the end of Ferid's troubles. I'm watching him when he turns and looks me right in the eyes. I cry in the police car and, later, at the hospital. The world feels grey, as though I've been deserted.

Ferid is brought to the emergency room. The police officers come back out to talk to me and ask me to stay outside, because my son doesn't want to see me. It's to be expected. More than one of them kindly reassures me, "You did the right thing, Ma'am. Stay strong." Everything has happened in record time. I stand there for a long while in the emergency room entrance. Nobody offers me a chair. I don't have anyone with me but God. All I can do is pray.

Catastrophic events can shatter memory, leaving us with only incongruous fragments. After the officers left, I was completely alone. I would come to understand that the most painful periods of life are when you feel most alone. They push us to adapt without anger because we have no other choice. I wait at the hospital for the entire afternoon. But all that matters is that my son is inside.

Eventually someone from the nursing staff comes over to explain the process. A psychiatrist will examine Ferid, and he'll only be kept at the hospital if the psychiatrist deems it necessary. If this ends up being the case, he can be kept for up to 24 hours by law. My son doesn't want to see me, he adds. He suggests I come back that evening with some of Ferid's personal belongings, some food and a toothbrush. I go back home, throw everything into a bag and return to the emergency ward. I meet with the psychiatrist, who tells me he hasn't been able to get anything out of Ferid. "He doesn't want to cooperate," he says. "I can't tell you anything. We'll keep him here until tomorrow, and another doctor will examine him."

I stay in the hallway until eventually Ferid agrees to see me. He's angry, and tells me I've humiliated him by forcing him out of his home in handcuffs, that I'm harassing him. "You're hurting me," he adds, talking about me and his father. "Leave me alone!" I blurt out my questions: How are you taking care of yourself? Do you have enough money for food? Your rent is your entire paycheck... We're worried about you. You never go out anymore. You never visit us. What's going on? Ferid doesn't answer. I realize the distance between us has become a gulf. Angry, yet lucid and very logical, he tells me point blank that I can do nothing to help him with this. He's aware that he has been isolating himself; it's something he's been battling for a long time. "I'm working on it," he tells me, "but I want to do it on my own." From his point of view, it's us, his family, who are hindering and harming him.

"I need some kind of minimum contact with you, Ferid. I can't live without that. Please give me at least that, to help me get through. Just to see you. I won't ask you for anything else. I just want to see you," I say, making a movement, I think, to take him in my arms, but he jerks away. So I go back to stand by the door. He softens a bit, hearing me explain how painful it has been for us. How we've missed him and lived in constant fear of never seeing him again. He asks me what exactly I want from him, at that moment.

"We want to make sure you're not suffering from some kind of illness." I don't want to be more specific than that, saying "illness," not "mental illness" with all its connotations, knowing anyone in his shoes would have reacted the same: insulted and judged without warrant, weighed down by the negative associations that all forms of mental disorders carry, including rejection and exclusion.

It takes generations to build awareness and change our collective consciousness. Mental disorders, diagnosed or not, hold a stigma that weighs on already-burdened shoulders. So I took care to explain how concerned we were as gently as I could. I referenced my own experiences with depression, a black hole that came with its fair share of social stigma. Society has a higher tolerance for depression even though there's still stigma attached. While it is a heavy and difficult thing for others to watch, people suffering from it still live and operate within the same reality. They know there is a problem and don't need anyone to throw it in their face or shame them. They manage on their own. At the end of the day, it's manageable.

All other forms of mental illness fall under the domain of the shamans of so-called Western medicine. Those who claim to have decoded the mystery of brain function. Which still is not fully proven.

Ferid got straight to the point. "What do you think psychiatrists do?! Did you stop to think for a second that, no matter what I say, they'll stick me in some sort of category? That's how this works. All that will happen is I'll walk out of here with a label."

I didn't know what to say. It was already late. So I said goodnight, told Ferid he could call me if he wanted to, at any time.

As I left, I remember him saying, "OK, I'll just tell them what they want to hear. If that's what I need to do to get out of here."

Monday, back at school. My mind is in two places at once, split between work and waiting for the doctors' verdict. I never use my cell phone at school, but that morning, I have it in my hand, and wait for a free moment so I can call the hospital. The psychiatrist I speak to calmly relates the results of the psychiatric report. "I spoke with your son. He's an intelligent, lucid young man. His thoughts seemed coherent. I could tell he is completely aware of the situation. He recognizes the difficulties he's experiencing, but is determined to overcome them on his own, in his own way. He's looking into ways of managing things. His solutions are not necessarily those a doctor would advise, but he wants to try to follow his own path, and we should take into account the way he wants to handle things." I let out a sigh of relief.

"What can we do to help him?" I ask.

"He needs support in terms of his material needs," the psychiatrist answers. "My advice would be to help in that way. Respect his decisions. Build trust by being present and patient with him."

Words couldn't express how thankful I was. For this break in the clouds. I thanked God, and life. And I resolved to follow the doctor's benevolent advice to the letter. I met with Majid and we established strict rules for how we would interact with Ferid. From that moment on, I'd no longer ask him about his projects or suggest solutions. It was time to accept Ferid the way he was and make peace with the rest. If I wanted to maintain contact with him, I needed to earn his trust so that he would open the door to let me in.

We decided all together—Ferid, Majid and I— that we'd see each other once a week, for everyone's benefit. I accepted that I'd have to stay at the doorstep. We talked a little and I'd hand him a package of food and some money. There was still no question of physical contact. But a hopeful ray of sunshine had entered my heart, and maybe his as well. Before leaving I thanked him for having me over and held back my tears till I reached the street. That's all a parent needs to be able to sleep at night: to see their child alive.

6. Starting Over

I kept my promise. I visited often and chose my words sparingly. "I love and respect you. I'm here, no matter what. I'm not judging you. I accept you just as you are. Thank you for opening the door to me." I tried to rebuild and nurture our relationship without forcing things. I was grateful for this small amount of contact.

Listening to other people tell us what to do can sometimes be a good thing, but it's always best to trust your heart and your gut. Ferid and I were no longer afraid of hurting each other. We were two adults on a path to reconciliation. His strength and restraint shone a light on my flaws, and I stepped down from my parental pulpit to stand next to him as an equal—to this man who had something important to teach me.

Majid and I slowly gained back Ferid's trust, to the point where we suggested he move closer to us, into a nice little apartment with reasonable rent. Love is the most impressive monument one can build, far greater than citadels, castles and empires. Once solidly constructed, it cannot be surpassed, can never be destroyed. In the end, everything crumbles and is forgotten. Absolutely everything. Except love. Love transcends reason. So our small amount of happiness began to produce little miracles.

We were there when he needed us, and no more than that. Eventually Ferid began opening the door and I'd step inside without saying a word. I'd buy pastries and bring them by, knowing he loved them, and then leave on tiptoe. I showered him in love. Time turned backward. I was fixing things, beginning to heal. I was learning things I'd been blind to before. And my teacher was Ferid. A wise man, a simple man. An upstanding person who was both capable and patient. Someone who had survived on minimum wage for numerous years, the rent and bills swallowing everything and leaving him almost nothing to eat.

Parenting is not an art that can be studied. We learn to be parents on the job, and we do our best. Life is sometimes generous and gives us the chance to fix our mistakes and become better people. "Please call me, whenever you need help," I told Ferid.

7. First Signs

It's September 2009. We've gotten into the habit of chatting at the doorstep. About anything and everything. Ferid has been talking to me about metaphysics and spirituality—interesting topics. He calmly asks if I think our souls are immortal, if there is an afterlife. These kinds of subjects fascinate me, and I give him my thoughts. I talk about my beliefs, why I believe we're here on this Earth and how, as I see it, we are more than mere organisms destined to be devoured by worms. It's a pleasure to listen to him talk, even if I find some concepts harder to grasp because they're so abstract. It seems as though Ferid has been delving into certain areas of quantum physics and the kind of deep thinking it demands. I can see the attraction of studying subjects that are beyond most people's comprehension. I'm not here to judge though. I've always had an open mind and been willing to discuss anything. I see this as an attempt for Ferid to socialize. Something he's in need of. Sometimes we converse for over an hour this way. I leave feeling lighter.

One evening when I stop by to bring him a little bag of pastries, Ferid seems feverish and exhausted. He tells me he hasn't been able to sleep. The same thoughts have been keeping him awake and it's taking a toll. He tells me about a mission he needs to be part of but that he's scared he won't be able to succeed. There's a worrying level of distress and anxiety in his voice. He confides to me that he belongs to an organization dedicated to safeguarding humanity, which is at the mercy of powerful agents working behind the scenes for a powerful secret organization: the Illuminati. Ferid says this brotherhood has been puppeteering governments for centuries now, and we are unaware our lives are in peril.

Over the next few days, I do some research to better understand Ferid's delusion. Online articles on the Illuminati abound, and there's room for any and all interpretation. It's difficult to sort fact from fiction. It's fertile ground for all sorts of conclusions. As someone with their feet planted in reality's muck, what worries me are all the pitfalls of the system in general. But for Ferid, who has slowly been cutting himself off from the world, the real issue is something different: the covert influence of powerful secret societies planning to take over the world. Right now this is his fight—and what gives his life meaning. It would be futile, even disrespectful, to try to shatter that reality. Some two years later when his brother casually mentions the Illuminati, Ferid tells Adam to drop it, that it's all nonsense. I came to understand that our truths shift according to our needs of the moment.

But that night after talking to Ferid on his doorstep for four hours, I responded to my son's distress and destitution as calmly as possible. "I know you want to be part of the mission," I told him, "but to do so you need to be in good shape. You need to take care of yourself first." I didn't want to deny him his reality, even if it didn't correspond to his situation. But he couldn't see that. He was lost in what he believed. I tried to act as a mirror to help him calm down and come back to himself.

I suggested that we go to the emergency room together, assuring him that he could trust the doctors to help. He told me he needed to go for a walk to first clear his head. I went back home. Two hours later the phone rang. It was midnight. It was Ferid—he was ready to go to the hospital.

8. First Hospitalization

> "We don't listen to them during psychotic episodes. We don't want to engage in their delusions."
> –Resident doctor in psychiatry, Montreal Jewish General Hospital, 2009

I drive Ferid to the Jewish General Hospital. We sit in the car outside emergency and talk for two hours. He knows he's not doing well. More than anything he just needs me to listen. I'm patient and attentive through it all. He tells me about everything that's been tormenting him—things he believes are related to a mental health disorder. Would he have come here of his own volition if he didn't? This is the state of mind he's in when the triage nurse interviewed him alone while I'm in the waiting room. I can picture him sitting there calmly answering the nurse's questions. Ferid describes his condition and admits he has been having suicidal thoughts. They hospitalize him immediately.

The medical report would say that Ferid felt suicidal after realizing he couldn't be part of a mission to save humanity. The resulting distress brought on symptoms that included disorganized thinking and delusions.

From that moment I'm plunged into a world of chaos where I'm a shadow, a rag doll, someone afflicted by association. Between work, managing the house, being a mother to my youngest son and being present for Ferid, I start running out of steam.

I go to the hospital's psychiatry department the morning after Ferid is admitted. I'm not allowed to see my son but I speak to the health professional who's caring for him. She tells me quickly while walking down the hall, "Your son's having a psychotic episode." She didn't even stop. For most people "psychotic episode" conjures up all sorts of prejudice and clichéd assumptions about mental disorders. I'm well aware that there's something wrong with Ferid, having experienced the dark recesses of depression myself and felt its repercussions, but I'm not ready for this. I can't quite process the information. It hits me suddenly, and hard. I feel like I'm stepping into a foreign country where I don't understand anything. Announcing a diagnosis to a parent this way shows a complete lack of respect.

I parsed the verdict that had just been casually thrown my way—information that is anything but casual. Did I ask questions? Yes. Which ones? I can't remember. I felt helpless, frozen. I was so frightened that I didn't think I'd be able to manage the uncertainty.

Since I have no further information from any of the medical staff, I turn to the internet and search for a definition of "psychotic episode": a period characterized by delusions and hallucinations that—thank God—may only be temporary. I desperately cling to this definition. If I've understood right, it's a symptom, not an illness. But a symptom of what? I keep reading and find that it can result from an underlying mental illness (a term I've now replaced with "mental health disorder"). The list of mental disorders jumps out at me from the screen—it's a long one. I start reading the symptoms of each. It all proves dangerously subjective since it relies on a degree of personal observation. Lines blur between disorders, and symptoms overlap. Reading it fills me with panic and a feeling of powerlessness, yet I feel justified for being skeptical and also somewhat in denial. Denial is the first line of defence against collapse.

You can find anything on the internet. I start to see that information has been cut and pasted here and there, grabbed and re-used on different websites, with virtually no sources or author names. Who should I trust? These psychiatrists, operating under the banner of silence? Some of whom, worse still, practically tell you that certain side effects—such as emotional indifference[1]—are the fault of the disorder and not the drugs. Other sites, like santé. canoe.ca,[2] go so far as to claim that schizophrenia is incurable, contradicting a substantial body of research that is often inaccessible to the public.

Under these conditions, it doesn't take much for parents who are distraught by the situation and paralyzed by the lack of information to pressure loved ones with a mental disorder to follow medical advice to the letter. In these contexts, the white coats are seen as nothing short of saviours.

I need to get a handle on what's happening so I can understand what we're up against. At first I'm deeply distressed. I still feel lost, and I retreat into myself. But I fight off despair, even though it's difficult. I know one thing: my son is hurting. Best-case scenario, it's major depression. Most of the symptoms Ferid has described to me are ones I've experienced myself, including suicidal thoughts, which I managed to overcome, outmanoeuvre, confront and understand over time. I accept that my son is sick, that he is having delusions, talking about suicide, and desperately wants the suffering to stop. I know what that's like. I spent a long time medicated. I also know that left untreated, depression eats away at you until there's nothing left.

Ferid's doctor made no mention to me about his real diagnosis—the actual name of his condition. We, his family, were kept out of the loop and completely in the dark. My son was experiencing psychosis they said: a loss of contact with reality that can be a sign of an underlying mental disorder or may just be temporary. I settled for this scrap of knowledge, somewhere between hope and ignorance.

I didn't come across the word "schizophre-nia" until months later, long after Ferid had been released from the hospital. Waiting alone in an Emploi Québec office, I saw it written on the social assistance application I was submitting for Ferid, for whom I was now the legal guardian. It knocked the wind out of me. I felt frightened and panic-stricken. I couldn't accept this death sen-tence. And that's exactly what it felt like: the kind of loss a parent experiences after being hit with the brutal news of their child's death. The world as I knew it collapsed. I was at a loss for words, moments before I was meant to submit Ferid's diagnosis to the Emploi Québec agent in charge of his file. My son was suffering from "that"! My eyes moved slowly across each letter of the lethal word. And then my mind shut down and tried to keep this thought out at all costs. I couldn't let the diagnosis get through. It was there like a sort of cancer, and I wasn't ready to deal with it. It took everything I had to anchor myself to the present. I was entering the first stage of grieving—denial offers protection. It's the wall we lean against to gather our strength so we can keep going.

As soon as Ferid was admitted to the hospital, I was informed that a resident doctor would be treating him. I ran down the hall to catch up with this young woman as if our lives depended on it to ask how they planned to help my son and about his chances for recovery. If there is one place the very concept of hope is practically non-existent, it is within those hospital walls. Doctors distill and deliver information in fragments as they run from place to place, eyes already elsewhere, accustomed to the sad but usual order of things. In the psychiatric ward, everyone is always running.

I don't remember seeing Ferid the day after his hospitalization, or the day after that. Did they let me visit him then? Or only once his condition had deteriorated? I can't remember. My memory holds a jumble of events that I still can't place chronologically. What I do know is that I went to the hospital after work to visit Ferid. I was told he had been placed in an isolation room, that the medication wasn't having an effect and he was talking about killing himself. Prescription drugs are like a club to the head, a way of knocking a highly complex biological being to the ground and gagging them. They either work or they don't; it's all or nothing.

They ask me to wait in the waiting room. I start praying. I get down on my knees and rest my head on the floor. I know the staff might open the door any moment and see me this way. Maybe they will make some connection with Ferid. It doesn't matter. I pray for myself, my family and my son. Did I see Ferid that night? I search my memory; I can picture myself there at the edge of his bed, encircled in light. Him silent; me depleted. Oddly it makes me think of an image of Vincent van Gogh in his tiny room sitting facing a window he'd brightened with his brilliant mind. Then

I see those white walls again, the bed bolted to the floor. The air is thick with silence. Silence is a remedy in desperate times when we feel completely powerless. Everything was created for a reason. These moments are precious because they signify the communion of what is universal: suffering.

The best ways we have found to heal individuals traumatized by life is to isolate, restrain and medicate them, under the pretext that they've lost all reason. We forget or pretend to have forgotten that there's always a part of the person that is still sane. It's this part of Ferid that allowed him to realize he was hurting and needed help. Nobody forced him to ask for help. When I urged Ferid to put his faith in the health system, I never could have imagined the kind of care he would receive. Never. Not in Quebec. I naively expected to find empathetic staff willing to listen, who prioritized the therapeutic relationship and communication and had long since cast aside antiquated methods. Then again, who was I to judge their methods? The first thing I did when I was finally able to meet with the staff was recount Ferid's history, in all its intricacies and complexities. It wasn't an easy conversation. At that point, I still believed the staff would incorporate this information into his formal therapy in some way.

That was my introduction to the world of the severely suffering. A large ward containing closed rooms with beds bolted to the floor and large barred windows to prevent suicide attempts. Under lock and key. Some patients remained isolated in their rooms while others who showed improvement moved freely about the common area. That evening my son and I sat in contemplative silence, just happy to be near one another.

Ferid stayed for a few days in the psychiatric ward, where the other patients often smiled or shyly greeted me in passing, moving aside as I walked towards the common area. I watched them with a wounded heart. It was unjust that life had taken their health, and often at such a young age. I'll never forget that place. Of all the time spent in institutions when my children were ill, this was the coldest and the greyest, with the terrible impassiveness of the hospital staff in the background reminiscent, if I'm honest, of a prison. What kind of healing could possibly occur in such a place?

Sitting at the edge of Ferid's bed, I listen to him talk feverishly. He's terrified as he describes the horrors of his delusions. He repeats certain details, insisting on their vileness, recounting them to me so he can be rid of them, can distance himself from them, with me as his witness, as he begs for my help. He holds his head in his hands trying to choke out the words, trying to free himself from the magma that burns inside him and won't let him rest. He's a prisoner of his own torturous thoughts, and he needs a reassuring presence at his side. This overwhelming need to speak to someone, to cling to another person, to let out his fear and empty the terrifying ideas from his mind are so vital, so urgent, that all I can do is hold his hand and reassure him. I can feel how much pain he is in. And I can feel him relax as soon as I gently pat his hand and whisper that everything will be okay, that he will make it through this. For the moment, my physical presence and my words have a soothing effect.

This approach—the act of listening—should be the preferred method of communicating with a person who is suffering to build the trust so crucial to recovery. But instead what's offered is this: isolation and a chemical cocktail we know almost nothing about. We muzzle, contain and constrict to stem the flow. To resolve things. But what about the underlying problems? I tried to understand the logic behind treating these people with so little human decency and compassion and failing to engage in the most basic introspection. Here is what Jean-Claude St-Onge says in his book *Tous fous?*:

> By reducing everything to biology, psychological distress is dehumanized and social misery is naturalized. Biopsychiatry removes individuals from their contexts: they no longer have a life story and are reduced to symptoms, abstractions. [...]
>
> If an individual is sick, it is due to an endogenous defect, a biological flaw they are likely harboring. We thought this would destigmatize mental illness [...]. This perspective depicts the individual

as a passive player stripped of personal agency. They are a prisoner in their own body. But humans are not passive when faced with external aggression and their psyche has the capacity to adapt to make these forces less harmful, or even to halt their effects.[3]

According to Ferid and the numerous other patients I've spoken to, self-awareness—the rational side—is always there. It's observing the situation. And yet the healthcare team working to stabilize my son's condition with medication never bothered to involve him in his own recovery process; for instance, by giving him a say in the decisions that concerned him. They failed to take into account any of his goals for the future and never bothered to ask why he'd refused to partake in the arts and crafts or sculpting sessions. The authors of the book *Je suis une personne, pas une maladie !* (I'm a person, not an illness) note the importance of the patient's role in the recovery process:

> Empowerment is a concept Dr. Gaston Harnois, former psychiatrist at Montreal's Douglas Hospital, ardently defends and promotes. It essentially set the tone for a mental health policy in 1989 and remains a guiding force for mental health services.[4]

Bill 120, passed on September 4, 1991, reaffirms that the guidelines governing the provision of health and social services in Quebec prioritize the individual requiring those services.[5] In other words, the user is their *raison d'être*. While this is clear in the Act, it's not the case inside hospital walls.

I asked the resident doctor why my son had been left alone without someone to listen to him, and the response I received was completely barbaric. "We don't listen to them during psychotic episodes. Our priority is to stabilize them."

"Why?"

"We don't want to engage in their delusions."

The violence of medical interventions causes additional trauma that hinders any kind of therapeutic relationship. During a psychotic episode, patients are no longer considered to be people suffering but as cases to be stabilized. They are later encouraged to partake in therapy where delusions have no place or significance. And yet these delusions are an integral part of that person's experience and important in their treatment. Isn't listening to the person in pain a form of therapy in itself? Trauma caused by mental health disorders is so trivialized it is often brushed aside. It's an added weight to an already heavy load of experiences, fuelling a vicious cycle. Refusing to give a patient experiencing psychosis their preferred treatment is not only unethical, but it also perpetuates the systematic stigmatization and dismissal of the patient.

Twist of fate

The day after Ferid's death, his two psychiatrists would finally take the time to listen to me. They were trying to better understand what had driven my son to take his own life. During the meeting I told them that listening to a person during an episode of psychosis was not incompatible with a biomedical approach to treatment; that the two complement each other. Ferid had tried in vain to make his voice heard. He'd tirelessly repeated, "I know I have to work with them and follow the treatment plan, but I'm also a person. I have a right to my say in things."

It was too late for my son, but I hoped the two doctors would finally be able to grasp that their approach (stabilize first, talk after) wasn't what Ferid had wanted. Many psychiatry professionals argue that it is futile to talk or argue with a person experiencing delusions and hallucinations. But that's misleading, as it isn't as much about communication as it is listening. The goal is not to show the person suffering that they're wrong but to show empathy, which is something foreign to psychiatry practice.

On October 26, 2011, the AQPAMM (the Quebec association for parents and friends of people living with mental illness) held a conference where Dr. Danielle Thibault put forward the following hypothesis, which in my opinion sums up the response of an empathetic, logical person:

"Why would a delusion have meaning? Because a delusion is a speech act—an act of human discourse, the same as any other speech act." Again, it's not a question of discussing the person's truth or reality during an episode.

Thibault goes on to explain the benefits of listening:

> In engaging in my practice of listening, I've become convinced that it is in many if not most cases the best solution. And in all cases, listening *first*.
>
> My experience as a listener has also taught me that listening means being attentive to the person's attitude and emotions far more than the content of their words. To what they're experiencing and feeling far more than what they're saying. The goal of listening is to help the person articulate their problem, understand themselves and build awareness, to then arrive at their own solutions, where possible.
>
> Why wouldn't listening to someone experiencing delusions have, at least in part, this same effect? One thing is certain: real listening is a source of compassion, and compassion always has a positive impact.[6]

It should follow that an approach centred around listening is vital from the start of hospitalization, especially when the patients and relatives express a wish for it. While it might prove reassuring for families that the health system decide what interventions should occur, to the point of going the legal route to assert its power, failure to offer support not covered by protocol—such as that of a psychologist, priest or loving friend—is downright nonsensical and borders on psychological cruelty. It didn't take me long to realize that what is in fact happening is that the patient is being subjected to an act of control. Stabilizing the patient means eliminating the symptoms of their mental health disorder, medicating them and sending them home as soon as they seem to have collected themselves.

How can we ask a patient to trust people who won't listen to what they have to say about their own treatment? How can we ask them to come in as an outpatient to learn how to reintegrate into society, when the hospital is where they have been the most alone in their suffering, isolation and double depersonalization (i.e., imposed by their condition and a system that is meant to help)? Prescribing based on trial and error, then releasing patients as soon as they tick all the boxes for what's considered "normal" is far from an achievement. The underlying problem hasn't been addressed.

The relationship between patients and their health professionals is based on a power dynamic that is legitimized by an omnipotent psychiatric machine. Human contact is kept to a minimum. The patient is the case and the family, by extension, the root of the problem.

9. Electroshock Treatment

"Take your pills or lose your bed."
–Ferid's psychiatrist, Montreal Jewish
General Hospital, 2009

Ferid's condition has been deteriorating for the past few days. He's been talking about ending his life so the pain will stop. He's being kept in isolation. His psychiatrist says the drugs are no longer working, that we need to switch gears and consider other options. She gets straight to the point. For the first time, the team is all in the same room to talk to me about a more draconian solution: electroshock treatment. Ferid's doctor has already spoken to him about it, and now my son wants to know what I think. I'm completely stunned. I'd thought this practice was banned, relegated to psychiatry's dark past. I get the same response from the staff whenever I ask questions: they stand stony-faced in front of me and list off the benefits with, of course, no mention of the treatment's side effects or long-term effectiveness. No one can provide me with brochures or other literature to make an informed decision. It's surreal. I feel as though I'm in a different era. The stark violence of this new reality is overwhelming. And the staff expect me to trust them blindly and just sign the form! My instincts tell me otherwise: that my son is in real danger.

One Flew Over the Cuckoo's Nest starring Jack Nicholson comes to mind. I'm suddenly very afraid of the hospital, these people and their practices. We feel weighed down by pressure from the treatment team. My son and I discuss it. I have no information to go on. I can't bring myself to imagine my son being wheeled into their care on a stretcher. I have an ominous feeling that they're keeping important details from me. They have deliberately failed to tell me how many rounds of treatment there will be, the details of the procedure, or its side effects and success rates. And Ferid is suffering so much that he's put himself entirely in my hands. "I trust you, Mom. You decide."

I don't waste any time. An online search for shock treatment used here and elsewhere turns up enough disturbing information and testimonials from traumatized patients that I refuse. While the practice has changed its name to the more in vogue "electroconvulsive therapy" (ECT) to dissociate from its dark past, the facts remain the same. Many doctors report a near absence of reliable studies that prove its long-term effectiveness. The repercussions to memory and cognitive function are, however, well documented by scientists and patients of all kinds. In an article titled "Psychiatry's Electroconvulsive Shock Treatment: A Crime Against Humanity," Lawrence Stevens, J.D., who has defended psychiatric patients, demystifies the treatment and explains what it entails. Citing a large number of psychiatrists who condemn its use, Stevens reports the negative after-effects on patients, including, in some cases, suicide.

> Some psychiatrists falsely claim ECT consists of a very small amount of electricity being passed through the brain. In fact, the 70 to 400 volts and 200 to 1600 milliamperes used in ECT is quite powerful. The power applied in ECT is typically as great as that found in the wall sockets in your home. It could kill the "patient" if the current were not limited to the head.[1]

In this same article, Psychologist Norman S. Sutherland notes that ECT often elicits high levels of stress in patients. "There are many reports from patients likening the atmosphere in hospital on days when ECT was to be administered to that of a prison on the day of an execution."[2]

Physical damage caused by ECT was discovered following autopsies carried out not long after Italians Lucio Bini and Ugo Cerletti invented the treatment in 1938. These include "cerebral hemorrhages (abnormal bleeding), edema (excessive accumulation of fluid), cortical atrophy (shrinkage of the cerebral cortex, or outer layers of the brain), dilated perivascular spaces in the brain, fibrosis (thickening and scarring), gliosis (growth of abnormal tissue) and rarefied and partially destroyed brain tissue."[3] Karl H. Pribram, emeritus at Stanford University's Neuropsychology Laboratory, observes the extent of the physical damage inflicted on the brain when ECT is used. He writes, "I'd rather have a small lobotomy than a series of electroconvulsive shock. [...] I just know what the brain looks like after a series of shocks, and it's not very pleasant to look at."[4] Neurologist Sidney Sament defines electroconvulsive therapy as "a controlled type of brain damage produced by electrical means."[5]

The health technology and intervention agency AÉTMIS, mandated by Quebec's health and social services ministry to assess the use of electric shock treatment, notes in its 2003 report that, "The medium- and long-term impacts include adverse effects on memory as well as other cognitive functions. [...] In cases of schizophrenia, the amount of evidence as to [ECT's] effectiveness is very slim, despite more than half a century of use to treat this condition."[6]

The non-profit Action Autonomie has been organizing an annual event in Montreal for the past twelve years in protest of shock treatment. One of their committees, Pare-chocs, notes that the treatment is making a comeback. "In Quebec, we've gone from 4,000 ECT sessions in 1988 to over 8,000 in 2003—a 100 percent increase. Two

out of three patients receiving ECT are women."
It adds that, "ECT is oppressive, violent and
undermines the integrity and dignity of the individuals. [...] Vulnerable people serve as guinea
pigs for this experimental treatment."[7]

Families must seriously weigh the pros and
cons of electroshock treatment by asking for comprehensive information and by taking the time
to think it over before signing the consent form.
Family members often have limited resources
and may be uninformed, suffering and lacking
support themselves. Feeling helpless, they may
place too much trust in the medical staff who they
believe will act in their best interest. These professionals do not have tangible evidence as to the
benefits or long-term risks of this treatment and
are protected by the associations they belong to.

Ferid and I refused to sign the consent form
that would have allowed the treatment team to
"speed up his stabilization." No, my son wouldn't
be submitting himself to this kind of torture.

Going off medication

My interactions with the healthcare team had
become tense, bordering on hostile. I saw everything, recorded every detail, and my notes were
corroborated by my son's disillusioned observa-
tions. Ferid was experiencing psychosis, but that
didn't mean he'd lost all reason. His speech was
coherent for the most part. Both of us felt the

same way about numerous events that took place in this psychiatric ward. I'd naively believed the staff would get him back on his feet, but what they cared about was that he take his pills—"or lose his bed," as his psychiatrist would tell him—and that the medication take effect.

It is generally the patient who decides to stop medication, since they are the ones experiencing its side effects. Some psychiatrists are quick to attribute these side effects to the condition itself, even if this is not the case, as I'd later learn. In his book *Tous fous?*, St-Onge explains further:

> [During clinical trials] observations led to questions concerning the effectiveness and tolerance of antipsychotics. Twenty to 40 percent of patients are treatment resistant to first generation drugs and nonadherence varies from 41 to 55 percent.
>
> As for the newer drugs, after four months around half of patients do not respond to treatment with Risperdal and Zyprexa. [...]
>
> A double-blind controlled [CATIE] study commissioned by the NIMH [National Institute of Mental Health] and published in 2005 showed an astonishing discontinuation rate of 74 percent. [...]
>
> These numbers were confirmed by a 2012 study on new antipsychotics (Abilify, Seroquel, Zyprexa and Risperdal), which followed 332 patients over two years. The rate of discontinuation hovered at about 80 percent: 51.9 percent due to side effects and 26.9 percent due to a lack of effectiveness. Half of patients stopped their medication within six months.[8]

When he was admitted to the hospital, Ferid was feverish but very hopeful about recovery. By the time he came out, this hope had been completely obliterated. He quickly became aware of the wide gap in equality between the patients and staff, and little wiggle room for those at the bottom, i.e. the patient or their family. We're far from an ideal partnership between treatment team, patient and family. Far from access to a personalized intervention plan, where the patient's opinion actually counts for something. There's a complete disconnect between the propaganda on hospital websites and the reality within hospital walls, a gulf filled with lies and hostility.

10. Reality on the Ground

I had been anxiously awaiting the family meetings I'd heard so much about, which would direct us to resources outside the hospital to help with long-term support. But these meetings never took place. I remember asking a nurse where parents could go for help, and all she did was point to a poster taped to the wall behind her for the Quebec association for parents and friends of people living with mental illness (AQPAMM). In terms of guidance and support, this is certainly a quick, cost-effective solution for the mental health system!

When Ferid was first admitted, I had been under the impression that the psychiatry department organized information and support sessions for family members. But just when we needed them the most, they were no longer available. How can access to such crucial services be so erratic, so dependent on political agendas and health ministry budgets?

As the head of a single-parent family, I was primarily the one keeping track of everything going on with Ferid, dividing my remaining time between my full-time job and the thankless role of mothering a pre-teen son. I added evening meetings at AQPAMM to my long to-do list, attending them when I wasn't too exhausted.

While this association does offer its members support, a space to talk, meetings and conferences, the services did not meet my family's specific needs. Different nights would focus on different topics, addressing, for example, mothers with teens struggling with bipolar disorder or borderline personality disorder. They did not, however, cover the struggles of a single mother whose son had schizophrenia. I couldn't help but compare my own situation to theirs and almost envied their lot, which I judged to be less of a burden than my own.

I also joined the province's schizophrenia association, the Société québécoise de la schizophrénie, which offers support to people living with a mental disorder through activities led by peers and their families. Yet many of my questions remained unanswered even after they were voiced in the community space, especially those related to medication. The association also organizes lectures for members. They can be useful, assuming our health care system actually offers access to the alternative resources and therapeutic approaches praised so highly by specialists.

Health service blind spots

We're told that families need to be equipped, informed and engaged to fully support someone with a mental disorder. But this is absolutely not the reality on the ground, where things are a tangled, disjointed mess. Our experience, and that of numerous other families, seems a truer image of what things are really like; this is evident in the results of a vast consultation with fifty organizations across 12 regions of Quebec on issues related to diagnosis, psychiatric medication, access to psychosocial services and different views on mental health.[1]

The consultation—led in preparation for a forum held in Victoriaville on April 15, 2016, on the theme "youth and mental health"—gathered near-identical statements and proposed solutions from the participants.

Here is a brief summary:

- We must fight against drug-based solutions to the problems our youth are facing using a comprehensive approach to intervention and promoting youth empowerment. This should be considered a social issue.
- Access to information and public services must be guaranteed.
- Alternative mental-health approaches and resources must be recognized and developed, so that youth have real choices.

- Training must be offered to youth, parents and professionals working with youth.

My experience lacked crucial elements from the very start of Ferid's hospitalization: a complete absence of support for our family, a failure to communicate basic information about Ferid's medication, the disengaged social worker, a lack of coordination between hospital services and external resources—and that's just for starters. It should not be the responsibility of family/friend support associations and mental-health advocacy groups to fill the gaps in the health system.

11. Home from the Hospital

"Any drug without toxic effects is not a drug at all."
–Eli Lilly, founder of Eli Lilly and Company, one of the world's biggest pharmaceutical companies[1]

Ferid's health did eventually improve. We prepared for his return home, developed a new routine and supported him in his recovery. We were directed to a day hospital for follow-up. His psychiatrist prescribed Zyprexa (a second-generation antipsychotic) and Clomipramine (a tricyclic antidepressant). We were not given any information about the side effects or risks of either drug.

Since Ferid was no longer a minor, we couldn't access information that would have allowed us to better support him—information about the powerful antipsychotic he had just been prescribed, for instance. The drug's adverse effects, which are well-known and documented, can be fatal. I have no idea whether the psychiatrist took the time to discuss the side effects of the two medications and how to manage them.

I first learned that Ferid was taking these drugs on an Emploi Québec form. It hadn't ever crossed my mind that medication could be toxic, other than in the case of an overdose. But every drug is toxic to some extent.

Big pharma's questionable practices

Terence Young launched an investigation into the drug industry following the tragic death of his daughter Vanessa. At age 15, Vanessa died after taking Prepulsid, a dangerous drug prescribed to treat vomiting. In *Death by Prescription,*[2] her father, a former member of parliament, uncovers drug industry practices that jeopardize the lives and health of citizens to the profit of shareholders. These are not accidents or isolated cases; they are the result of deliberate actions. Young speaks to Dr. Neil Shear, who notes that "the most comprehensive study on adverse drug reactions was done using U.S. statistics by Lazarou, Pomeranz and Corey from the University of Toronto published in the *Journal of the American Medical Association* in 1998. They believed it was higher than a hundred thousand a year in hospitals." Young goes on to find evidence that "perhaps 39 percent of all adverse drug reactions in hospitals are *preventable*. Assuming 10,000 hospitals a year, if we acted, we could save perhaps 4,000 lives a year in hospitals."[3] And that's not counting the number of deaths outside hospital walls, either due to a prescription or dispensing error, or to accidental overdose.

One example among many: my daughter believes that her baby, who is one month old at the time, is in pain after undergoing a minor surgical operation under local anesthetic, even though he isn't writhing in discomfort and doesn't seem to have a fever. She gives him a dose of Tempra, an oral acetaminophen solution for pain and fever relief. My daughter isn't the first parent to administer this kind of medication to her kids without pausing to read the fine print. I grab the box and note the warning, in bold: an overdose can lead to potentially fatal liver damage. On the health site Ressources Santé[4] there are no fewer than 25 side effects listed for this drug, including several severe ones: back pain, bleeding, fatigue, fever and chills, allergic reactions, respiratory difficulties, swelling of the face and throat and liver damage. I tell her, "Breastmilk is the best remedy for this sort of thing!" But in her mind, I'm overreacting.

An overdose of Tempra can cause serious liver damage and even death; administered to a month-old baby, how do the benefits outweigh this long list of side effects? Especially since it's impossible to know what a baby is feeling. Many infants have died without known cause, their death often attributed to the notorious Sudden Infant Death Syndrome. After reading through the long list of Tempra's side effects, what parent would then click on the link, "Are there other precautions or warnings for this medication?" It either makes you want to cross your fingers and hope for the best or throw the bottle in the trash! We need to take the initiative to inform, and thereby empower, ourselves so that we can protect our lives and the lives of those around us.

Before I lost my son, I never knew that taking medication could be dangerous—very dangerous, in fact. It is doubly revolting to discover that an industry meant to help people has such a hold over governments and their agencies so they can turn a profit.

12. Road to Recovery or Dead-End?

It takes remarkable ineptitude to push young people with mental health disorders to participate in activities they've neither chosen nor been consulted about. Peer support worker and consultant Luc Vigneault agrees. Vigneault works at the Institut universitaire en santé mentale de Québec and is well known in mental health circles for his workshops and lectures. He believes that the trauma experienced during psychiatric hospitalization scars patients and hinders the therapeutic relationship. And he would know; he struggles with a mental health disorder and once attended a treatment meeting where the staff predicted a dim future for him, in front of his family.

> Once I left the hospital the stigma weighed heavy, and I became a prisoner of my medication's iatrogenic effects, i.e., the effects *they* had caused. I soon grew accustomed to the revolving door effect, caught in a vicious cycle of trips back and forth to the institution. On one of my trips to the psychiatric ward, I received the following decisive prognosis: "You're done," then to my family, "He's

done. He'll never be able to work or have a social life or be romantically involved."[1]

Luc's healthcare team believed that his mental illness—diagnosed as schizophrenia—was incurable. But his family and friends didn't give up on him. They fought for the hospital to change its treatment approach. His file was transferred to another team specializing in lost causes. Their credo was "Rather than fight to eradicate the symptoms of an illness, we advocate for treatment based around a person's life goals [...]. Only the individual is equipped to identify these goals. There's always some part of us that's still rational."[2]

Psychiatrist Marie-Luce Quintal, head of medicine at the Centre de traitement et de réadaptation de Nemours (the Nemours treatment and re-adaptation centre) in Quebec City, and professor at Université Laval's Faculty of Medicine considers recovery to be a personal journey.

> [It is] an experience that means different things for different people [...]. Healthcare professionals must be highly adaptable as they share their knowledge with a person who arrives with a different set of knowledge. It means the individual not only has a say in the decisions made about them, but that they have knowledge no one else does. [...] They know what they like, [...] what's important to them, what makes sense and what they absolutely cannot afford to lose. Above all, they alone can find their path to recovery.[3]

Let's take the example of homelessness and mental illness. Psychiatrist Marie-Carmen Plante notes that, over the past 30 years, there has been a substantial rise in the number of people who are homeless and living with chronic psychiatric problems, chronic alcoholism and/or serious substance addictions who are in search of food and shelter, especially during winter cold snaps. They arrive at Emergency, where they are not treated specifically by psychiatric services. Inspired by the work of numerous doctors, including Leona Bachrach,[4] Dr. Plante made a list of problems encountered daily by her team of clinicians and psychosocial workers:[5]

- Barriers in accessing psychiatric care
- Fragmentation of mental health services
- Lack of liaison and communication
- Defensive and inflexible division of mental health services
- Limitations of approaches and treatment of comorbidity and polymorbidity[6]
- Increased use of biochemical treatment to the detriment of therapeutic relationships
- Deinstitutionalization due to austerity measures, such as budget cuts and fewer hospital beds
- Successive mental health policies that translate to few changes on the ground
- Lack of planning for the period following homeless patients' release from care

- Inadequate understanding of the realities and specific needs of people with mental health issues who are living on the streets when preparing treatment plans, etc.

According to psychiatrist Georges Nauleau, staff working with individuals experiencing homelessness must adopt an individualized approach.

> Despite how the many people we meet on the street and in emergency shelters show signs of numerous psychological disorders, often but not always alongside addiction (alcohol, drugs, etc.)—from psychological suffering linked to precarious living conditions to the most severe of mental disorders—it's impossible to generalize as to the life experiences or trajectories of these individuals.[7]

Dr. Nauleau notes the importance of patience when working with someone experiencing homelessness, regardless of their mental health history.

> We need to understand the pace and parameters of their world—this person who is asking so little—whether that world is marked by psychosis or not, and consider what kind of relational distance the person is comfortable with. Otherwise the crucial and often long work that has been undertaken to find an approach and build a connection for a strong therapeutic relationship, or simply one of support, must be redone.[8]

Outreach is a proactive approach that involves visiting the spaces homeless individuals occupy and taking actions based on respect for their realities and choices. Will this be the method used at the day hospital where my son is referred, after his release from the psychiatric unit? I'm hopeful. The psychiatrist who takes on Ferid's case and the staff member who works with him are more open. I feel that I'll be able to communicate with them. I come with Ferid to the first few appointments of the eight-week program. Ferid's doctor urges him to continue his medication and encourages him to participate in the discussion groups and other activities aimed at reintegration.

I still have a copy of the weekly program. Looking at it now, I realize it fails to mention the group discussion topics, or the type of activities planned. Let's think about that for a moment: in addition to having no say in the outpatient clinic programming, patients don't even have the proper information to decide whether or not they want to attend these voluntary sessions. Would you travel to the clinic under these circumstances, when all signs point to a dead end?

It might well be that the program suits certain patients, but my son is shy. In his most difficult moments, he would rather keep to himself to avoid speaking up or causing conflict. He resists from the inside. I still encourage him to go. "Just getting out of the house and taking the metro will do you good," I tell him. I'm unknowingly breaking my promise not to impose decisions on him. I've lost confidence in my judgment and in my ability to act based on my values and principles.

Eventually my son, infuriated, is direct with me. "Mom, listen. Here's how the meetings go: someone in a white coat sits in front of me with a form that's essentially the same as the one at Emergency. They go through a list of questions and check off my answers. Is this what recovery is supposed to be?"

Since there's no coordination or information exchange between family members and the care team, there's no way for me to argue for the program's benefits. Looking back today, it's clear to me why he didn't want to attend. At first Ferid had had an almost unwavering confidence in his clinicians, but that was greatly diminished by the end of his stay in the psychiatric ward. We both realized that neither he nor I had a say in things. They made the decisions, in our best interest. What would break Ferid's trust in the medical system for good was the damage his medication would cause.

13. Drug-Free Treatment

Everyone has their own notion of recovery. Patricia Deegan, who has schizophrenia, fulfilled her dream of becoming a psychologist—but she did so without telling her doctor fearing that he would discourage her. Today she's a researcher and lecturer. Deegan has conducted a meta-analysis of seven long-term studies on recovery. According to her results[1] the recovery rate for people with serious mental illnesses, including schizophrenia, ranges from 46 to 68 percent. A bearer of hope, Deegan maintains that people diagnosed with mental illness are strong; they are not merely passive victims. She also maintains that therapists able to see their patients' active, flexible, strong selves support this more empowering view. Deegan describes recovery as "a process, a way of life, an attitude and a way of approaching the day's challenges." She continues:

> Recovery does not refer to an end product or result. It does not mean that [we] are cured. In fact, our recovery is marked by an ever-deepening acceptance of our limitations. But now, rather than being an occasion for despair, we find that our personal

limitations are the ground from which spring our own unique possibilities. This is the paradox of recovery, i.e., that in accepting what we cannot do or be, we begin to discover who we can be and what we can do.[2]

The first few days after Ferid is discharged from the hospital, we come together as a family again. My son is happy to see us all together, and he decides to take us out to eat. We talk about the future. We had dreamed of such gatherings and promise to make it a habit. Family becomes very important to Ferid again. At his own pace, he resumes his life—but a life very different from the one he'd led before his hospitalization. He rediscovers the special bond he had with his younger brother, a bond they had both missed so much all those years that we silently and internally bore Ferid's suffering. The two of them have fun playfighting on the sofa, throwing cushions at each other. Once they even broke an ill-fated lampshade that had been set down nearby and laughed as they told me that it didn't belong there anyway! Moments like these are a godsend.

But the side effects of Ferid's medication cast a shadow over everything. We're not seeing an improvement in his health but a continual deterioration. Obeying the doctors' sacred orders, we nevertheless urge him to bear the unbearable. We keep hoping he'll recover, but what's happening is the opposite. And it's heartbreaking to witness.

Ferid soon begins to have difficulty sleeping. He gains weight. His movements slow down; he drags his feet. He can't stop shaking. Even seated, he compulsively taps his thighs with his fingers. His mind is elsewhere. He has difficulty speaking and stares off into space so silently that it scares us. His face is frozen as if he were wearing a mask, his handsome features hidden behind stiffened muscles. Sometimes he paces the living room, smiling aimlessly and muttering to himself. He is suffering physically and mentally. It's so terrible and distressing to see him like this.

How can you ask someone so knocked out by medication to make the insurmountable effort necessary to leave the house and attend day treatment activities at the hospital? It is a vicious circle that the psychiatrists seem to either fail to grasp or to deliberately ignore. How do they expect their patients to cooperate when they know what agony they're in? Do they really believe that their patients don't make the connection between their side effects and their doctors' willful blindness?

Ferid had lost all quality of life. Would we have to wait weeks, or even months, to hope to see an improvement in his health? Adjusting his dose and adding new medications only made things worse. He couldn't take it anymore. But in an effort to listen to me, he kept focusing on deadlines. I can still hear him, muttering with glassy eyes, "Two more months, Mom. But I won't be taking these pills my whole life." His doctors hadn't told him how long his treatment would last, nor had they broached the topic of side effects. My son certainly would have told me if they had, if only to justify his decision to stop taking his pills.

Even though I asked Ferid's psychiatrist at the outpatient clinic about his medication, he was no more talkative than his inpatient colleagues. What's more, the family support that we'd so hoped for was limited to phone-call reminders for appointments. Talking to the nurse in charge of his file, I tried to explain how Ferid's weariness and lack of motivation prevented him from leaving the house. She didn't bat an eye, blaming it all on his illness. Why not visit him and help him in his own environment? I asked. She firmly refused, "My job is to offer my services to your son, not to you." As if I'd asked for help cleaning the house. Citing her job's limitations and working conditions, she didn't want to leave her comfort zone and seemed unable to imagine acting any differently in order to build a meaningful therapeutic relationship with her patient. In the end all she did was increase the number of appointment letters she sent, which Ferid no longer even bothered to open.

Then one day my son decided to stop taking his medication. It was simply the final outcome of a medical approach that was doomed from the start: "Mom, they're nothing but pill pushers at the hospital!"

The Scandinavian and Finnish examples

Medication-free psychiatric treatment is now a reality in Norway as a result of the lobbying and joint action of five user organizations.[3] In 2011 the Norwegian Ministry of Health began by sending out a letter to regional health authorities recommending that they create a few beds for psychiatric patients wanting drug-free treatment. The letters were routinely ignored, so the Ministry of Health turned their recommendation into a requirement in 2015. "Many patients in mental health care do not want treatment with medication," the Norwegian Health Minister writes. "We must listen to them and take this seriously. No one will be forced to take medication as long as there are other ways to provide the necessary care and treatment."[4]

In nearby Lapland, Finland, another, even more humanistic approach has had real success in treating schizophrenia.[5] Open Dialogue is based on the principle of open conversation, without secrecy or hierarchy, and values the patient's voice in their care and treatment.[6] Jaakko Seikkula, professor of psychology and founder of the Open Dialogue method, places the utmost importance on his patients' words: the patient is not only the bearer of meaning, they should be the very starting point of the therapeutic relationship. According to Dr. Seikkula, anyone can suffer from psychosis.

Any of us could experience a psychotic problem. It's a response to a very difficult life situation. If I'm faced with a situation that's very stressful for me, I might start to hear voices, for instance. And those voices or those experiences include things that have previously happened in my life. [...]

At the first meeting, I can't understand what their words mean. But later on, step by step, I start to realize that, actually, they're talking about something that has actually happened and this may be the first time that it's become possible for them to have words for it. It's a kind of metaphoric way of speaking of experiences that they didn't have any words for before.[7]

Open Dialogue therapists recommend taking as much time as necessary before delivering a diagnosis. They also recommend being clear and specific in one's explanations when diagnosing someone with schizophrenia, because the diagnosis is terrifying and may cripple the patient and their sense of initiative and creativity.

Meeting spaces for Open Dialogue therapy are chosen by the patients and their families. The healthcare team is able to do home visits, where the patients can express themselves freely in their natural environment without fear of legal consequences. If the patient would rather meet elsewhere, sessions can also take place somewhere such as a coffee shop. The therapists work as a team and discuss their impressions and reflections openly in front of the patients and their families, who are placed on an equal footing. In his documentary on the topic, psychologist and director Daniel Mackler notes that while these practices seem very reasonable, they're quite different from current mental healthcare practice in the United States.[8]

The Quebec and Canadian healthcare systems have a lot to learn from other models. It is up to us, as users and caregivers, to push for a paradigm shift.

14. Three Years of Remission

When one person falls ill, their whole family is generally affected. This is particularly true when it comes to mental illness. We spoke little of Ferid's schizophrenia. I couldn't talk about such a severe mental health problem without fully understanding it and what caused it. Right up to the end of my son's brave journey, we feared the word. Ferid himself uttered it only once or twice. I will remember one of these times until my dying day: "Mom, do you really think I'm schizophrenic?" I evaded his question with a vague answer, my eyes lowered. I was ashamed that I'd failed to love my son enough to protect him from this evil. I wasn't able to deliver this blow—to confirm a truth I myself couldn't accept.

Grieving parents all have something in common. We've all wished that we could have died instead of our children. We would have liked to take their place; it's easier to suffer yourself than to watch your child suffer and not be able to do anything about it. In truth, we grieve twice over.

For other kinds of illness, science is able to demonstrate natural or physiological causes.

Mental illness is diagnosed only on the basis of its symptoms, classified by the *Diagnostic and Statistical Manual of Mental Disorders* (DSM), which has been published by the American Psychiatric Association since 1952. Yet the number of mental illnesses listed in the DSM has soared over the past 25 years. As Jean-Claude St-Onge notes in *Tous fous?*:

> Things have changed dramatically since the publication of the first edition of the DSM in 1952. Not only have behaviours that were once considered more or less normal been added to the "bible" of psychiatry, but the number of them has exploded. Since the Second World War, the number of mental disorders in the DSM has increased from 106 in 1952 to around 400 in 1992 and will increase even more with the publication of the DSM-5 in 2013.[1]

St-Onge's book contains a wealth of information on the world of psychiatry, its internal wars and blunders, inflexibility toward innovation and dangerous contamination by the powers of the pharmaceutical industry. This is an industry that sees a potential mental illness in all of us and doesn't hesitate to sell—lawfully and with full knowledge of the facts—ineffective, dangerous and even lethal products, including antipsychotics, antidepressants and sleeping pills. Thanks to St-Onge's exceptional work and the work of others, such as Terence Young,[2] I was able to not only make the connection between my son's side effects and his prescription medications, but also found confirmation of many of the questions I'd been asking about the workings of the health-care system. Sadly I learned more than I wanted to know.

Once Ferid's pills were back in the bath-room cabinet where they belonged, he gradually emerged from his fog. He started to lose the weight he'd put on while medicated and became present again. He spent less time with his imaginary friends. A smile returned to his beautiful face. His step was lighter, and he started to join me on errands. In the evenings he was radiant and optimistic. That was enough for us.

Remission takes time and patience, but we live in a society where everything must be constantly moving. Too often we forget that we're not a character in a comic book or the hero of a Hollywood film. We compare ourselves to others and measure our success against theirs. We prove that we're employable and able to make money. We adjust to society's expectations. Should our right to be different and our right to free will be subject to societal normalcy, which serves its own needs and not those of individuals? In a group there will always be people who can work and others who can't succeed on all fronts. To aggressively push the most vulnerable among us to be independent helps no one—neither patients nor healthcare professionals. Rather, it has the opposite effect, generating an often-justified mistrust of an increasingly less humanist system. Sincere respect for people suffering from mental health disorders, and for their rights, calls for so much more.

15. Zyprexa

"A not insignificant percentage of Quebecois are functionally illiterate, and most of them are medically and pharmacologically illiterate."
–J.-Claude St-Onge, *L'envers de la pilule* (The darker side of pills)[1]

I consistently cite Zyprexa when talking about pharmacological illiteracy because I still feel guilty about not realizing how much suffering it was causing Ferid—suffering that his psychiatrists attributed to his illness. Driven by fear and worry, we pressured Ferid to continue poisoning himself to avoid a relapse. I can still see my son slumped on the sofa, staring vacantly or pacing around the room, completely cut off from us. Akathisia (or restlessness), indifference, weight gain, excessive fatigue, hallucinations, sleep problems: Can a drug that's supposed to prevent psychotic episodes so incapacitate a person? Is that the price we have to pay?

As I began reading more and more, I not only realized the extent of my ignorance, but also the ignorance of the ruthless institutions that manage our health as though it were a common commodity. I'm realizing that my son, who was swallowing down one of the most harmful second-generation antipsychotics, is one among innumerable victims of a corrupt system firmly in place all over the world.

The Zyprexa trial

Zyprexa (olanzapine) is a second-generation antipsychotic released in 1996 by Eli Lilly, the tenth largest pharmaceutical group in the world in terms of revenue. In 2007 it was estimated that this ostentatiously marketed drug had been or was being consumed by more than 20 million people, bringing in 4.7 billion dollars per year for Eli Lilly. Yet between 2005 and 2007, more than 28,000 claims were filed in the United States against the company for failure to provide information on the drug's side effects—diabetes and obesity in particular. To avoid public trials, the company settled out of court in 2005, offering an average financial compensation of US$90,000 to complainants.[2]

Around the same time, French whistleblower Elena Pasca noted that there were also "other charges against Lilly, starting with a shareholder complaint due to losses resulting from its conduct: namely, creating the illusion of a problem-free medication and encouraging investment when the company knew about, and tried to conceal, the drug's adverse effects."[3] Still according to her, the American government also filed a complaint against the pharmaceutical company, accusing it of being behind "too many unjustified prescriptions, and therefore expenditures, by advertising Zyprexa for uses beyond marketing authorization."[4]

In July 2008, New York judge Jack Weinstein held that the extent of the problem was rather due to the moral bankruptcy of US regulatory agencies:

A large part of the legal problems attributed to Zyprexa, if they exist, are arguably due to the failure of the responsible federal agencies to prevent abuse. A jury might credit evidence that the government and its responsible agencies did not adequately ensure that the available knowledge of pharmacological efficacy and dangers, to the extent they can and should have been known, were rapidly communicated to prescribing doctors, third-party payers [...] and even patients. Compared to its peer agencies in other parts of the world, the United States Food and Drug Administration (FDA) has arguably failed consumers and physicians by overrelying on pharmaceutical companies to provide supporting research for new drug applications; by allowing them, through lax enforcement, to conduct off-label marketing; by acquiescing to industry pressure on drug labels; by not requiring doctors—the main line of defense against misusing prescriptions—to be adequately informed; and by leaving information dispersal and control largely to industry-influenced medical journals and non-governmental associations.[5]

While it was protected by a patent, Zyprexa was sold at 100 times the price of perphenazine, a first-generation antipsychotic. Yet today the commonly held view is that these more costly second-generation antipsychotics are not any better than their first-generation counterparts. In other words, they are new products with no added value. J.-Claude St-Onge devotes an entire chapter to Zyprexa in his excellent book *Les dérives de l'industrie de la santé* (The Abuses of the Healthcare Industry).

A double-blind controlled study conducted by the National Institute of Mental Health (NIMH) and led by Dr. Jeffrey A. Lieberman compared [Risperdal, Seroquel, Geodon and Zyprexa] to perphenazine in 1,493 patients suffering from schizophrenia. The authors of the study, which was published in September 2005 in the *New England Journal of Medicine*, concluded that "the efficacy of the conventional antipsychotic agent perphenazine appeared similar to that of quetiapine [Seroquel], risperidone [Risperdal], and ziprasidone [Geodon]." Olanzapine (Zyprexa) was most effective in terms of the rate of discontinuation [64 percent compared to 74–82 percent for the other four]. However, it has been linked to serious adverse effects such as substantial weight gain and increases in glucose measures, both of which increase the risk of developing diabetes.[6]

In addition, internationally recognized psycho-pharmacologist Dr. David Healy noted that "olan-zapine [Zyprexa] and risperidone [Risperdal] have in fact a greater number of suicides, deaths and suicide attempts linked to them in their pre-licensing trials than any other psychotropic drugs in history."[7] Starting in 2005, whistleblowers such as Dr. David Graham, Associate Director of the FDA, were raising alarms about Zyprexa and Riperdal—both of which can cause diabetes, heart problems, and even death—being prescribed for off-label uses, such as treating dementia in elderly people and behavioural problems in children.[8] These off-label uses, though the FDA knew about them, may have led to an additional 62,000 deaths per year: a true massacre.

In spite of all this, doctors continue to prescribe Zyprexa with impunity in Quebec today. No one informed our son or us, his family, of these risks. No psychiatrist ever advised him to use Zyprexa sparingly or temporarily or to try alternative treatments. It was not for want of asking his psychiatrists for their opinion.

Health is not simply the absence of symptoms or the ability to meet the criteria of normalcy; it is much more. The patient's self-esteem, an essential part of their recovery, is the first thing to suffer and the last thing to be taken into account in psychiatric hospitalizations.

Long-term use of antipsychotics

In the absence of appropriate psychosocial support, long-term use of antipsychotics reduces the chances of recovery for people with psychoses.

The majority of clinical trials are short-term—no more than 12 weeks—and are carried out on patients who are not representative of clinical practice in terms of age and comorbidity (i.e., the presence of one or more disorders associated with the primary illness). These shortfalls prevent us from confirming whether any real differences exist between different antipsychotics. As Jean-Claude St-Onge reports in *Tous fous?*, the National Institute of Mental Health (NIMH) organized a six-week trial to test the effectiveness of antipsychotics on 344 people in 1961. While significant improvements were seen in 75 percent of patients on antipsychotics compared to 23 percent of those on placebo, three years later, patients given the placebo were less likely to be rehospitalized than patients in the first group, who frequently wound up in the emergency room—a trend they termed "revolving doors." While researchers report that the symptoms of medicated patients tend to persist and worsen, Joanna Moncrieff, a psychiatrist at University College London, notes that psychotic episodes tend to diminish on their own for most people.[9] More recent studies have come to the same conclusions.

In the wake of the new study by Dutch researcher Lex Wunderink, it is time for psychiatry to do the right thing and acknowledge that, if it wants to do best by its patients, it must change its protocols for using antipsychotics. The current standard of care, which—in practice—involves continual use of antipsychotics for all patients diagnosed with a psychotic disorder, clearly reduces the opportunity for long-term *functional* recovery.[10]

In this *Mad in America* article, Robert Whitaker compares Open Dialogue in Finland with the results of two long-term studies: Martin Harrow's study of 145 people with schizophrenia followed over a 15-year period with Lex Wunderink's study of 103 patients followed over seven years.[11] At the end of Harrow's study, the recovery rate for patients off antipsychotics was 40 percent, compared to 5 percent for patients who had maintained antipsychotic drug therapy. In Wunderink's study the group that had discontinued or reduced their antipsychotics had a recovery rate of 40 percent compared to 17 percent for the group that had maintained their usual dose.[12]

Open Dialogue therapy goes even further by recommending that antipsychotics be used as late as possible in a first psychotic episode, as appropriate psychosocial support and the selective use of benzodiazepines[13] may mean that the patient can recover without ever having to take them. With this selective use of antipsychotics,

Open Dialogue has produced the best long-term results in the developed world.

The findings of these studies are consistent with the conclusions of Professor Joan-Ramon Laporte and his team at the Centre Midi-Pyrénées de PharmacoVigilance, who have found that medication fails to modify the pathophysiology of the illness, in addition to causing serious side effects.

> Continuous and prolonged exposure to antipsychotics produces cerebral atrophy and irreversible impairment of cognitive function. The incidence and severity of the side effects on the extrapyramidal system and metabolism increase with the duration of treatment.
>
> In spite of this, manufacturers and numerous clinical practice guidelines recommend that psychotic patients be treated indefinitely. This contradicts the results of meta-analyses of clinical trials, which have shown that intermittent treatment results in fewer relapses. Antipsychotics lead to a dependency requiring that treatment be tapered off progressively to avoid withdrawal symptoms (discontinuation syndrome).[14]

The responsibility of prescribing physicians

Everything I ended up learning about antipsychotics is consistent with my son's experience with Zyprexa: the medication induces the very symptoms it is supposed to fight. Sudden cessation then causes symptoms that are mistaken for the illness returning. Nearly all literature available online, including from pharmaceutical companies, conflates the symptoms of schizophrenia with prescription drug side effects, thereby shackling the patient to a lifetime of medication. And indeed, there is a danger of confusing the symptoms of schizophrenia and the side effects of antipsychotics: the former include disorganized speech, hallucinations and delusions; the latter paradoxical effects that can cause tardive dyskinesia, upper motor neuron syndrome (affecting voluntary motor skills), diabetes, increased triglycerides, weight gain, brain atrophy and, in some cases, delusions, hallucinations and suicidal thoughts.

In his book *Deadly Medicines and Organised Crime*, Peter C. Gøtzsche, physician and co-founder of the Cochrane Collaboration, maintains that "psychotropic drugs don't fix a chemical imbalance, they cause it, which is why it is so difficult to come off the drugs again. If taken for more than a few weeks, these drugs create the diseases they were intended to cure. We have turned schizophrenia, ADHD and depression, which were often self-limited diseases in the past, into chronic disorders because of the drugs we use."[15] Some psychiatrists use this very reason to justify the long-term, uninterrupted use of antipsychotics.

What about prescribing physicians? It seems they are no better informed than we are, blindly following drug representatives who are willing to dangerously filter or distort information about these drugs so they can turn a profit.

There is no shortage of testimonials. Shahram Ahari, former Eli Lilly drug rep who mainly promoted Zyprexa, speaks eloquently on the topic. In a video Ahari openly recounts the ploys used to influence doctors. It is a testament to Eli Lilly's absolute cynicism.[16] How many doctors make the time and effort to verify information they receive from drug representatives? After all, doctors are the ones who will be held accountable when there's an accident due to a drug's side effects. The truth of the current situation is a call for us to open our eyes and wake up from our consumer slumber.

16. Schizophrenia

"If you talk to God, you are praying; if God talks to you, you have schizophrenia."
–Thomas Szasz, psychiatrist and thinker in the anti-psychiatry movement

And now we come to a topic that continues to be contentious in scientific communities: schizophrenia. How do we define it? What causes it? What do we tell people who have it, and how long do we wait? No one at the hospital ever explained these things to me—this will, unfortunately, be my refrain throughout the book. In my son's case, I'm not sure if he received any information related to his diagnosis.

Ferid and I almost never broached the subject. He knew that he was suffering from something, but didn't accept his diagnosis. As his caregiver, I was supposed to understand this humiliating word, but had only ever overheard it in the hospital halls. The first bits of information gleaned here and there, mostly from the family support association AQPAMM, led me to believe it was an illness of the brain with multiple complex causes and factors, most of which remained a mystery.

The Wikipedia entry, various websites and scientific literature all describe the illness as a curse. In his book *Saving Normal*, Allen Frances, an American psychiatrist who worked on the revisions to DSM-4 (*Diagnostic and Statistical Manual of Mental Disorders*) but became a vocal critic of the DMS-5, writes:

> Schizophrenia is a useful construct—not myth, not disease. It is a description of a particular set of psychiatric problems, not an explanation of their cause. Someday we will have a much more accurate understanding and more precise way of describing these same problems.[1]

In the 1980s, renowned American psychiatrist Thomas S. Szasz, a key figure and radical thinker of the anti-psychiatry movement, argued that schizophrenia, the "sacred symbol of psychiatry,"[2] does not exist as a mental disorder in itself. According to Szasz, the diagnosis only reduces the person to a victim. His opinions did little, unfortunately, to prevent the label from being used politically, socially and medically on millions of people whose only fault was to experience psychosis.

I was so convinced of being a bad mother that guilt had become a second skin. When you're trying to get perspective in this kind of situation, a pat on the back and a reminder that it could happen to anyone is not enough. It's no exaggeration when I say today, looking back with clear eyes: no other

diagnosis could have made me feel so ill, so powerless. It destroyed part of my soul; it made me dream
of death as a possible deliverance. Let's not forget,
though, that the label was above all something my
son had to carry with him wherever he went.

Schizophrenia is a severe mental disorder
that, according to the World Health Organization
(WHO), affects more than 20 million people across
the globe.[3] In Canada, an estimated 1 percent of the
population lives with schizophrenia.[4] Symptoms
most often appear during adolescence or early
adulthood. High suicide rates among youth are
often connected to the label's stigma and its effect
on self-image and hope for the future, rather than
a perception that the disorder is incurable.[5]

> The mortality associated with schizophrenia is
> one of the most distressing consequences of the
> disorder. Approximately 40 percent to 60 percent
> of individuals with schizophrenia attempt suicide,
> and they are between 15 to 25 times more likely
> than the general population to die from a suicide
> attempt. Approximately 10 percent will die from
> suicide. [...]
>   Public misunderstanding and fear contribute
> to the serious stigma associated with schizophre-
> nia. Contrary to popular opinion, most individuals
> with the disorder are withdrawn and not violent.
> Nonetheless, the stigma of violence interferes with
> an individual's ability to acquire housing, employ-
> ment and treatment, and also compounds difficul-
> ties in social relationships. These stereotypes also
> increase the burden on families and care givers.[6]

Can we really go by these statistics? What kind of message are they sending? Rereading them now, I feel that the focus is once again on the negative impacts of the illness, eclipsing the rest: the individual's strength, resilience and rich and complex personality. Do people living with mental disorders have any say at all over their civil rights? Do hospitalized psychiatric patients receive adequate and respectful care in terms of what they want and don't want? Are they treated with safe, effective drugs that do not pose major health risks? Do they have a right to alternative treatment if they refuse medication? Do they have access to all the necessary information? Do the transitional housing placements offer a safe and abuse-free environment? Are there governmental bodies monitoring conditions in these supervised establishments? What preventative measures are in place to keep people safe and off the streets? Do we have the ability to adequately inform the public about the realities of living with a severe mental disorder without further stigmatizing the people living with them? What kind of support can we offer caregivers?

An article in *Time* magazine dated July 6, 1992, called schizophrenia "the most devilish of mental illnesses."[7] How can we call an illness "devilish"? Even specialists can't agree on the definition.

In the Foreword to *DSM-II*, Ernest M. Gruenberg, M.D., D.P.H., Chairman of the American Psychiatric Association's Committee on Nomenclature and

Statistics, says "Consider, for example, the mental disorder labeled in the Manual as 'schizophrenia,' [...] Even if it had tried, the Committee could not establish agreement about what this disorder is" (p. ix). The third edition of the APA's *Diagnostic and Statistical Manual of Mental Disorders*, published in 1980, commonly called *DSMIII*, is also quite candid about the vagueness of the term. It says "The limits of the concept of Schizophrenia are unclear" (p. 181). The revision published in 1987, *DSMIIIR*, contains a similar statement: "It should be noted that no single feature is invariably present or seen only in Schizophrenia" (p. 188). *DSM-III-R* also says this about a related (so-called) diagnosis, *Schizoaffective Disorder*: "The term *Schizoaffective Disorder* has been used in many different ways since it was first introduced as a subtype of Schizophrenia, and represents one of the most confusing and controversial concepts in psychiatric nosology" (p. 208). [...]

The Third Edition-Revised (*DSM-III-R*), published in 1987, says a diagnosis of schizophrenia "is made only when it cannot be established that an organic factor initiated and maintained the disturbance" (*DSM-III-R*, p. 187).[8]

As a leading critic of DSM-5, Dr. Allen Frances has denounced a tendency to see mental illness at every turn. In an article in *Psychology Today*, he cites a study that found that 81 percent of children "had already qualified for one diagnosis of mental disorder" by the age of 21.[9] Dr. Frances also acknowledged responsibility for his role in fuelling three false mental illness epidemics (autism, ADHD and bipolar disorder), as J.-Claude St-Onge notes in *TDAH? Pour en finir avec le dopage des enfants* (ADHD? Let's stop drugging our kids).[10]

The toll on family

As soon as Ferid stopped taking his medication, he started feeling better. He made the decision to stop four or five months after his first hospitalization, in spring 2010. Then began to emerge from a zombie-like state. Today, I thank God he did. My son accepted the hand he'd been dealt with a clear head. And it's one thing I'm grateful for.

Ferid moved at his own pace. He never inconvenienced or attempted to harm anyone when he walked down the street. He was a gentle creature who didn't like being told what to do. When we'd suggest adding anything to his routine, he'd gently decline. "Later," he'd tell us, "when I'm feeling better." We became accustomed to hearing this. He attended holiday celebrations and birthdays, calm and gentle as always, and picked out the most thoughtful gifts. It made him smile to see us happy.

Our worries remained, however dormant. An added challenge was that I was the only parent and sole caregiver. My daughter had a life of her own, and lived 40 kilometres out of town. She had a husband and new baby—her first child.

Not being able to do anything for her big brother weighed on her, as did the little time I had to visit her, so she came to see us almost every week. I regularly declined her invitations to go to her home, under one pretext or another, even though she knew the real reason I kept saying no. When I would reluctantly agree to come for the weekend, I was always apprehensive, trapped in a vice of anxiety that inevitably turned to resentment at having to leave Ferid. It was a constant state of suffering. My work as a teacher, while it was demanding, also allowed me to compartmentalize different parts of my life and build up my armor. Though a teacher's workload is notoriously heavy, it alleviated my constant anxiety. The boys' father started visiting less often, for reasons we didn't want to say aloud. I suppose he had a hard time understanding and accepting the kinds of problems Ferid was experiencing.

And then there was Adam. He was starting high school, and the transition came with its own challenges: a new school, new environment, new friends, constant pressure from his teachers. The teaching staff soon pegged his bubbly nature and constant need to move as attention deficit hyperactivity disorder (ADHD). Our family doctor prescribed Concerta (methylphenidate, also sold under the brand name Ritalin) with a single but significant warning: the drugs might stunt Adam's growth. A lack of appetite was evident after the first few days—a bad sign from the beginning.

Aside from dependency, Concerta has a long list of side effects, including verbal tics, aggression or hostile behaviour, agitation, anxiety, nervous tension, lack of appetite or refusal to eat, hallucinations, signs of paranoid behaviour or depression, profound sadness, hopelessness, a feeling of uselessness, guilt, mood changes, risks to the heart and brain, growth suppression and weight loss.

Information varies online from one site to the next. For ample and accurate information, it is best to turn to solid scientific research on the subject.[11]

In the teaching world, I often hear colleagues or childcare workers causally make diagnoses about kids, even if the child in question has a minor problem that just needs personalized attention. Every time I try to get help for a student, I'm asked the same infuriating question: is the child medicated? It shifts responsibility onto the parents and also presumes parental fault.

Adam became a model student almost overnight, at least according to his teachers. He no longer disrupted the class, laughed, or made anyone else laugh. His grades improved. His weight plummeted. But we just had to accept that his growth would be stunted. I decided to stop his medication, bluntly letting his teachers and doctor know that if I had to choose between his grades and his health, the decision was obvious. And then Adam started playing soccer on a regular basis, and everything settled down. Each of us in our own way managed to overcome the traumatizing events we were living through. Adam was stoic when his brother died. He kept playing soccer, going to school and seeing his friends, but he also turned to video games as an escape, and his homework suffered.

Difficult times

Back then I'd arrive home late, where the housework awaited. Exhausted, I sought the help of a psychoeducator to help me manage my time and Adam's homework. It was a difficult period, with all the worries piling up. I was constantly questioning my approach to dealing with each of my children, unsure if I was doing too much, if I was leaving them enough space to live their own lives, whether I was a good enough mom, if I was present or loving enough. I was in a state of psychological distress.

At times I'd go out and wander through the streets to escape from my looming fear of a future I could neither avoid nor control. Most times I'd park myself in the corner of a café, often at Place des Arts. I'd go there to try to forget my sorrows and put off facing reality. I didn't like myself. I considered my life a failure and a disaster. I ruminated over the past, going over the darkest memories in slow motion in search of what might have led my eldest son, my baby, into such a dark, maddening place where no one could reach him. I couldn't forgive myself. I knew Ferid's childhood trauma, my unstable relationship with Majid, the repeated separations, having to leave his friends, the never-ending anxieties of a refugee family in its long search for asylum, and reaching his teen years and arriving in a new country were all significant factors in triggering his mental illness.

In a 2016 lecture on the effects of social determinants of mental health given at the Université de Sherbrooke, J.-Claude St-Onge notes:

> According to the biomedical model, mental health is completely isolated from people's lives, as if life circumstances and how we interpret them had absolutely no impact on behaviour and mood. Abuse and negligence, humiliation, bullying, grief and failure, poverty, social inequality, powerlessness, obstructions of freedom and desire, existential questioning, an inability to make sense of life's blows... It's the blind spot in biomedical thinking.
>
> Numerous studies have shown evidence of this. Children who have lived through trauma are 2.78 to 11.5 times more likely to develop a psychosis, and every additional traumatic event elevates the risk by 240 percent (2.5 times). An article in the *Archives of General Psychiatry* notes that youth who have been sexually abused by more than one person have a risk that is 1,400 percent higher of a schizophrenia diagnosis, which DSM-5 has rebaptized the "Schizophrenia Spectrum." Diagnosis of depression goes up almost 490 percent in the poorest households compared to the richest ones,

and children of chronically unemployed parents are 400 percent more likely to develop symptoms of ADHD (hyperkinetic disorder) than children of professionals. In comparison, the C4 gene—related to synaptic pruning during adolescence—may increase the risk of schizophrenia by 25 percent. Added to the 1 percent considered a baseline risk, this brings it to 1.25 percent. To put that in perspective, smokers have an increased risk of 1,900 to 2,900 percent of dying of lung cancer.

Despite everything, I found hope somehow. I looked back on my own struggles with depression that punctuated my life. When I think back, it's clear these periods of my life coincided with problems that proved far too much for me to handle or solve alone. But at the time I attributed the sadness and hopelessness to the choices I'd made and ignored the greater social factors. I was insecure, afraid of losing my job—a pattern that was well ingrained into our family's history. Added to that was a feeling of inadequacy, of being different, the "other" who does not possess the same rights. I was the Algerian woman on the side of the road. My years spent in Algeria had held mixed emotions and I'd brought that bitter aftertaste to Vienna where, arriving as a refugee, I was the ignorant woman who didn't speak German. It had made me want to disappear into the background, deeply ashamed that I was unable to offer my children a decent life.

The residue of this low regard for myself and inadequacy faced with life's eventualities shaped the truth I held about myself: that I was a failure. Thoughts of suicide became a salvation at times, and the only power I held over my life back then. In *La route de la dignité*, I wrote about how I pushed down my pain, holding it there with all my strength to prevent it from harming the people I loved. I'm a survivor, so I believed in the power of nature, the promise of resilience and, above all, I felt safe living in one of the richest countries on the planet: Canada. Never did I doubt for a single second that this was the right place to raise my children. I trusted it to be true.

I'd received the help of my local CLSC (local community health services centre) 20 years prior. I'd first contacted SOS-suicide, where they advised me to go out and take a walk until I could get help the next day. Eventually the CLSC in one of my favourite neighbourhoods, Notre-Dame-de-Grâce, had a multidisciplinary team take charge of my case. The whole team was present and ready to help, and I felt it. They let me talk. I described my mental state, how I couldn't keep going. The reasons were complex. It was the classic case of a struggling immigrant family. The long-feared rupture of a couple that had finally taken place. An 18-month-old baby who cried all night, eyes glued to the window where he saw his absent father in the faces of each passing stranger. Two teenagers whom I counted on too much. All on top of extreme poverty.

It was low regard for myself but also guilt, a lack of family support and the weight of taboos. I started considering the fastest way out. Ending it. But I couldn't imagine leaving my children motherless. Their love is what held me back. I thought of how much harm suicide can cause. I pictured them without me, carrying with them a deep hurt they didn't deserve. I might not have been worth much in my own estimation, but what would my death mean for them?

The CLSC provided help that worked. They assigned me a social worker and allotted me financial aid, since we were living below the poverty line. It wasn't a lot of money, but it paid for me to put Adam in daycare while I looked for work. I started taking antidepressants, which alleviated the major symptoms of my depression. Therapy helped me see things in a different light and find new hope for the future. Soon after, I found a small teaching contract two days a week. I slowly rebuilt my self-esteem and began to feel I had a purpose. Without the support and empathy of the entire CLSC team, I don't believe I'd be here today writing this. I took it for granted that the health care system in Quebec worked this way across the board.

The health professionals that I've had the chance to speak with about our experience paint a portrait of the psychiatric world as harsh, closed, inaccessible, terrifying... In a way, my son paid the price for my ignorance and trust in the system.

Schizophrenia is not incurable, nor is it fatal. Far from it! But the lack of personalized treatment that considers a person's uniqueness and their goals can prompt them to want to end it all.

17. A Rich or an Impoverished Life?

The common conception of someone stamped with the label of a mental health disorder is that they have an impoverished life, which is a baseless value judgement. In taking the time to get to know the person, in kindly lending them our attention, we surprise ourselves by revisiting our assumptions. No person lives an impoverished life because they have an illness. This belief would be an underestimation of our ability to adapt, and of human resilience.

I've worked with children most of my life. I've spent time with people of all ages, with all kinds of issues, and I've never presumed to think any two people are alike. Whether it's a hearing impairment, autism, a developmental disability, Alzheimer's disease, bipolar disorder, major depression, schizophrenia or something else. We are not an illness. We are people. And we are all different.

As part of my degree in inclusive education, I remember one practicum that completely shifted my perspective. It was in a class of around 20 young people aged 13 to 18, all with different profiles. Some students were autistic, others had developmental disabilities, others still had multiple disabilities. Their educational program had been adapted accordingly and each teen worked at their own pace, the teacher guiding them with unbelievably caring support. The class was full of energy and excitement, and I was surrounded by smiling students who were bursting with life. I'd learn that from one person to the next, lives can differ vastly, and that no two are quite alike.

The first few days in that classroom, I felt useless. What did these kids have to learn from me? What did I have to learn from them? After 20 years I can see they were the ones who had something to teach me: how to be a humble teacher—something I'm still working on.

Marc was a handsome boy with a sparkle in his eye. He was autistic, nonverbal, had a severe movement disorder and was difficult to approach. When I said hello to the students, I'd give him a little smile from across the room, and he'd immediately look away. I spent time with the students who accepted my presence and gave the others time to get used to me. After a while, most of them warmed to me. Even Marc seemed to be waiting for me to turn and smile at him every morning. But if I intercepted his furtive glance, he would look away. Then, something miraculous happened. During an outing at the park one day, he came up to me and took my hand.

From then on, Marc never left my side. Attachment. A bond. Something that can only come from a place of trust, which he confided with his undefinable intelligence. At a party, I watched Marc dance, jump, twirl, hug me and lift me up in the air, elated. I had tears in my eyes. I felt badly that I had to leave at the end of my practicum, and I was afraid for him. What would he think? His teacher, Pierre, could see how concerned I was. "How will he accept me leaving?" I asked.

"Don't worry, he will," was his answer.

Marc was adopted. His adoptive parents loved and cared for him in spite of his severe disability. While there is no doubt he had a disability, he was also a passionate, sweet young man who had so much to offer. We have no right to reduce a human being, in all their complexity, to the confines of our ignorance. Bright lives, like stars, are those that continue to shine in our memories long after they're out of sight.

18. Relapse

> "The parable of the believers in their affection, mercy, and compassion for each other is that of a body. When any limb aches, the whole body reacts with sleeplessness and fever."
> –Prophet Muhammad A.S.

It's December 2012. Ferid isn't doing well. He starts sleeping 20 out of 24 hours, perhaps a reaction to the greyness of the brutal winter that has been battering everyone and everything in the city.

He never complains, just stoically endures the pain. I can read it on his face though, and in his slow movements, in how his shoulders slump further and further down even though he's not yet 32. I can also see it in how resigned he is after countless attempts to rally us behind a vision of a fairer, healthier world where everyone can live together in their own uniqueness, at their own pace.

Often he talks to me when I'm in the kitchen about the benefits of the organic products he has carefully selected in health food stores and lifestyle choices that could improve his health. He argues for the power of simplicity and love's ability to heal, of acceptance in its broadest sense. His energy has been dropping. He soon abandons his basement bedroom for his brother's bed upstairs. We don't agree with this, but we tolerate it because it seems to do him good. Later Ferid would tell us he'd wanted to escape the loneliness he felt downstairs in his suite. Hadn't my daughter said as much about having his room down there? The lack of light and minimal contact with us didn't help things. But upstairs he didn't have the privacy he sometimes needed. When I offered to give him my room instead of his brother's, he politely refused.

Around that same time, my mind became fixated on the sudden disappearance of my mother, who was still living in Algeria. Two friends of mine had passed away three months apart, and I began worrying that I'd never see my mother again. Each new loss amplified my anxiety. For my own peace of mind, I decided to visit Algeria. Guilt often does not lead us to the best decisions. Should I have cancelled my trip and stayed with Ferid? The more I think about it, the more I believe the answer is yes. Could I have changed the cascade of events to follow? I can't say. Like during all traumatic periods, I can only remember the pain. When part of the body suffers, the whole body suffers. The same goes for families and their members.

Isolated, lonely and exhausted

My powerlessness proved so depressing that the only way for me to get through the days, one at a time, was to pray. I prayed to God every morning to show me the right path to get Ferid the help he needed. The fact that it was difficult to have people over to the house isolated us further: we couldn't have guests without talking about Ferid's illness, side-stepping the label for fear of frightening people or lying and evading the unspoken questions in their eyes.

We began living in a vacuum. I'd sought out support from various associations, but it wasn't enough. Most of my family was in Algeria. Ferid's grandparents, aunts, uncles and cousins kept sending invitations, but he always declined. He said he wasn't strong enough to be able to enjoy this kind of trip, and I understood completely. Managing his daily routine was already a feat.

Without realizing or being able to help it, I'd come to love Ferid far more than my other two children, as though my intense attention could work miracles. That kind of love is an antidote to enduring despair. I remember how torn apart with worry my parents were when my sister was diagnosed with celiac disease. For years they heaped care onto her while the rest of us pawed at them, starved for affection, praying that God would inflict us with some illness that would get their attention. In Abla Farhoud's novel *Le fou d'Omar*, I was struck by how well she depicts how mental illness affects a family.

> I detest this father. His father. A father who has six kids but eyes only for him, interest only for him, love only for him [...]. Our family became a hive, and this son its queen, the damned condemning us along with him. [...] Our thoughts, our conversations, our interests all gravitated around the brother we had to save at all costs.

An entire family bound by misfortune. A misfortune that had struck not one of the family but each and every one of us, as though there were no space between us, no breath possible that did not taste of it.[1]

Silence fills the house. We're afraid to speak. Everything is fragile. In class I alternate between crying and laughing. To hide how bad I'm feeling, I make jokes with my students, who are concerned to see me hunched over at my desk for long periods. I make up little worries they can easily understand. And dozens of different excuses to avoid the staff lounge at lunchtime. I need my break to cry, pray and make phone calls. I'm falling to pieces. My resources are depleted. And pain radiates from my mind, paralyzing my entire body. I can't keep going like this.

I use the intercom to page the principal. She's a particularly attentive, kind person. She finds someone to take over the class right away and brings me to a small room next door. I don't have the strength to hold it in any longer, don't have enough tears to dispel everything that has been building up for so long inside. Ferid's name tumbles out of my mouth. I tell her about his mental illness, without going into the details, and explain that he hasn't left his bed in two months. She takes me in her arms and hugs me tightly. She tells me to go see my doctor, and I do, that same day, and am prescribed two months of sick leave.

We had entered a tunnel. Ferid was exhausted and left his bed only once in a while. What could I ask of him? To see a doctor? To relive the same experiences and frustrations? I'd long since lost faith in the health system. What can we expect of a young man who is sick and beaten down? A young man whose expectations of the system he landed in three years prior were met with indifference, disdain, condescension and a lack of understanding? Who wasn't given the chance to get a word in, to learn about his illness and what it would mean for him? To whom no one had offered any real hope for recovery or alternatives to the hospital-imposed solutions? What was left of my son once he'd been given this label? All the unbending, dehumanizing medical interventions had both amplified and justified his mistrust in the health system.

We're waiting for a miracle. January 2013 is a dark month. We barely have room to breathe. We're living as though in wartime. Expecting disaster to strike at any moment.

An exceptional degree of autonomy

It's impossible to say when exactly traces of the illness first surfaced. When his health had started to deteriorate, while he was living alone without anyone's help, his strength carried him beyond what should have been possible, without affecting anyone else. During these three symptom-free years, my son had gone about his life all on his own.

The extent of this autonomy was astounding considering his resources. The autonomy of a survivor can in no way be compared to that of a healthy person. His meagre income at the time likely didn't provide enough to eat. Yet he never asked anything of anyone. He must have deployed all the resources in his power so that he wouldn't be a burden. He had a sense of pride, and so he wanted to make things as easy as possible for me. If he could see I was tired, he'd suggest we order pizza, or that he cook instead.

He knew his limits and respected them. Working would have meant going back to school. Studying would have required a physical and mental capacity that he didn't possess. And beyond the state of his health, he possessed something called meaning. The meaning of one's life is founded on the conviction that we each have a place on this Earth, that we are worthy, respected, and that we can be of some kind of use, no matter how small. This is the drive behind achievement. No one, myself included, really knew Ferid. But he had a life just as important as anyone else's, legitimate dreams, hopes and convictions. He had a lot of love to give and, at his most vulnerable, he would turn to others to be heard. For someone to listen. Is that not a cry for help?

The trip to Algeria

I remember talking to Ferid about going to Algeria. I told him how much we all loved him. Especially his grandmother. How she missed him. She'd been asking the imam at her mosque to dedicate the Friday prayers to her grandson and his recovery. When you believe in God, that faith helps you grasp at hope and multiply it. It helps delegate our powerlessness to the All-Powerful, offering the respite needed in order to live through what life throws at us. So we pray. We trust in the universe. We know that nothing is a foregone conclusion.

We all thought a short trip to the place Ferid grew up would do him good. "Come with me," I said. "You won't have to travel around much."

He flashed me his enigmatic smile, one that told me I already had my answer. It hurt. Because his illness had gained ground and all we could do was stand by and watch. I pleaded with him to reconsider.

"Come with me. You'll see, it would do you good to visit the place where you grew up, maybe you could even see some of your old friends."

"Another time... when I'm better."

Preaching to people who are very ill serves no purpose. It's almost obscene. He'd made up his mind. But he said to me, "When you get there, Mom, don't forget to bring the whole family together like this—two hands together with their fingers interlaced. Stand in a circle and love each other." Now, I keep his message for posterity. Two days before I left, Ferid relapsed.

19. Ferid, aka Jesus Christ: A Second Psychotic Episode

It's almost spring. Ferid has a second psychotic episode, but this time he seems calm, almost transfigured. He isn't plagued by hallucinations, or exhausted by delusions. He has regained his strength as though by miracle. He's radiant. He seems liberated, with an exhilaration gently filling him with life again. I've never seen him like this, and it makes me afraid. Not of him, but for him. He's not aggressive or threatening; his usual reservedness has shifted to a strange exuberance for life. I would have liked to enjoy this feeling with him, but I'm afraid he is in danger.

It's late in the evening, around 10 or 11. Ferid comes into my room to tell me he's found a solution to our problems. Outside, it's snowing. He motions to the spectacular sight through the window saying, "Mom, look. Look, Mom, everything's perfect! I'm here now. I'm Jesus and I'm here to look after you all. We can do anything. You don't need to work anymore..."

"Ferid."

"It's all over now, Mom. I can get you everything you need. I'm going to go out and walk around."

I'm distressed but I keep listening. Adam stands quietly behind Ferid, watching. What should I do? Ferid isn't a danger to anyone. He isn't threatening anyone. He's delirious. He turns to his brother and says, pointing at himself, "I'm Jesus... I'll look after you."

How can I help him? Help us? How can I prevent an accident? It's my first time witnessing Ferid experience a religious delusion. During his first hospitalization, which took place of his own volition, his symptoms had been different: disorganized thinking and an obsession over the mission he believed he was part of. This time he repeats quietly that he has reached a "higher state" while, in his eyes, we remain mere humans.

"Mom, listen. I'm your son. But you should know that I've evolved. I've reached a higher state. I've reached here," he says with his hand above his head to show me. I keep listening, hoping to calm him down. "You—you're right here. I'm higher up—here. I recognize that you are my mother, but I'm also the son of God.

I'm not equipped for this and I'm afraid. While I don't fully understand the stages of his illness, I follow his logic. It's a personal journey that I can't counter with reason. Is it because I'm his mother he has such a hold on my heart? With nothing more than love and intuition, I instantly grasp the deeper meaning of his message. He'd taken the spiritual path that suited him best, inspired by the person most significant to him—Jesus—and whose qualities he identified with: humility, simplicity, kindness, love and the ability to help others through his connection to the Lord.

"You're Muslim, Mom, but I've left Islam. Now I'm Christ, the son of God. I'm sorry."

"It's okay, I understand."

In my mind it's clear: everything he says is symbolic. His words transcend our usual notion of reality to convey a message about his personal quest for meaning.

"Is it a crime to say you're Christ?"

"No, it's not."

He would ask this same question at the hospital, and I would later find it in his writing as well.

"You won't have to work anymore, Mom. Out there in nature we have everything we need to survive."

"And what about the bills, Ferid? Who will pay them if I stop working?"

He looks at me for a moment, presses his palm against his forehead and says, "Ah! OK, give me some time. I'll think about it and get back to you."

We're still able to engage and talk to each other. When he leaves my room, I grab the phone to call the police. He sees what I'm about to do and begs me to stop. I get him to calm down a bit, but still manage to hastily place the call. The person on the other end asks whether Ferid is a danger to himself or others.

"No, but he has a mental disorder and is off his medication. I'm scared he'll get hurt."

Several police cars pull up in front of the house. The officers see that Ferid shows no signs of aggression. With the same fervor, he tries to rally them to his cause. One of the officers turns to me and says they can't hospitalize my son against his will, since he isn't a danger to himself or to us. I end up explaining that I'll be out of the province for several days and that my son will be alone in the house, without help. They ask Ferid if he's willing to come with them to the hospital. He says yes. We decide that it's better if I stay home. My other son, Adam, is standing there in complete shock. I'd almost completely forgotten about him.

The next day the whole family goes to visit Ferid. He's still in the emergency room, waiting to be transferred to the psychiatric department. He's upset, and he expresses his anger lucidly: "I might be rambling, but is it so bad to believe I'm Jesus?"

No one knows how to answer. Then we hear someone in the next room, another young man who is barely 20, gently and patiently explain the same thing. "I'm Jesus, Christ the Lord. I'm Jesus," he says. I look over at him with the wounded heart of a mother, full of compassion for both of them.

What primordial need, what underlying message do our children deliver to us through their suffering? Is it the hope they have poured into a spirituality that is so often repressed, that they avoid showing publicly for fear of being labelled a degenerate or fanatic? So many people transcend suffering through the figure of Christ, who is a powerful symbol in the eyes of two thirds of humanity; the reason must be that it makes sense to them. And since this is their reality and their path, not ours, we have no right to judge. Instead we should have the courage to cross that border separating our worlds and hold out a hand. We should recognize that what they're saying has meaning and respect that. This approach is integral to recovery. So in the end, I'm glad my son is claiming to be Christ rather than falling prey to the voices that terrorized him during his first hospital stay. .

I approach Ferid and remind him that I'll be away for a while. He sees my apologetic eyes and makes a gesture not to worry, assuring me everything will be fine. I feel overwhelmingly guilty that I have to leave him. I'll only be gone 10 days, but I meet with the ER doctors to ask their opinion. "His father and sister are here. You need a rest. We'll look after him—don't worry."

Building on the person's healthy side

One thing is certain: we never lose ourselves completely to illness, whatever illness we may have. There is always a healthy part of us that remains, that nurtures us. Ferid had three good years. During that time he lived a content life, relatively at peace with himself and others, thanks to a healthy lifestyle he'd cultivated. He had relied on his intuition, building on his strengths and accepting his limitations. When we'd suggest adding something to his routine, he would weigh it carefully before calmly deciding. We'd gotten used to this reality. During that period of calm, we lived relatively well.

I'm convinced that had he been provided care that respected what he needed and wanted and took into account his limitations, it would have supported his recovery, especially after the second hospital stay. Instead the healthcare team never offered treatment that considered his life goals, ambitions or wishes. The day program was the same: the staff established the activities, with no input from participants. Why would anyone want to go? Our ability to choose what's best for us is a clear sign of a healthy mind. Other than an eight-week program most patients usually never saw through to the end, as the staff admitted, no other recovery care was offered or recommended to us.

In 1993, psychiatrist and researcher at Boston University, Dr. William Anthony, defined recovery as follows:

> [...] A deeply personal, unique process of changing one's attitudes, values, feelings, goals, skills, and/

or roles. It is a way of living a satisfying, hopeful, and contributing life even with limitations caused by illness. Recovery involves the development of new meaning and purpose in one's life as one grows beyond the catastrophic effects of mental illness.[1]

Université Laval professor and researcher Hélène Provencher in Quebec City writes:

Recovery is defined here as transcending the symptoms, functional limitations and social handicaps of a mental disorder. This transcendence shows up through multi-dimensional transformations that require initiating personal, interpersonal and socio-political processes to create a renewed sense of existence.[2]

These definitions focus on the healthy part of the individual rather than on their limitations. Provencher notes that recovery involves everyone: the individual and the people around them—family, friends and neighbors—along with mental health services and the surrounding community. For recovery to happen, there needs to be a well-informed team of healthcare professionals coordinating efforts, people who are able to put aside their own points of reference and adapt to all kinds of situations. Instead of pre-determined programs, the recovery process should be carried out with the patient and their support network. Both times Ferid was hospitalized, the services provided were oriented toward one thing only: eliminating his symptoms. Period.

Ferid stubbornly maintained throughout his second hospitalization that he was the son of God with a mission on Earth, categorically refusing to take any medication he felt unnecessary. At least he was making his opinion known, expressing his anger, debating, communicating, laughing and joking; this was a side of him I'd thought we had lost.

It's March, the month he was born. His sister, who is four years younger, comes to visit. They walk down the hospital hallways talking. At one point they pass someone and Ferid says to them, "Hi, I'm Jesus, Jesus Christ." Then turns to his sister with a sly smile and complicit wink, "I embarrassed you, eh, Jasmina?" It's incredible how someone who has lost reason can shift from one world to another, from one reality to the next, in order to defend their right to inhabit that space. What tremendous mental and emotional dexterity, or whatever you'd like to call it! And all the while understanding that not everyone can grasp their experience—and how difficult that is.

20. Court Authorization for Treatment

Since Ferid refuses to take his medication, the medical staff takes its standard course of action: they ask us to give them permission to file a treatment order with the Quebec Superior Court. The document submitted to the court falsely claims that Ferid has been "verbally aggressive" towards his family, then goes so far as to state that they plan to administer his drugs by injection to counter any acts of disobedience.

Did we fully understand the extent of this decision we were about to make for Ferid? They never explained the details of his treatment, how it would help him or what the possible reprecussions would be. They banked on our ignorance. Instead of making an informed decision, we were guided by our fear of the worst.

Something vital to consider: the very notion of "dangerousness" is questionable. No court ruling can be entirely objective when the decision essentially depends on the doctor's opinion. In addition to forming their own assessment, this doctor is also influenced by third-party accounts and police reports. Yes, Ferid was experiencing psychosis, but he was not aggressive. The religious nature of his claims made sense to him, even if he wasn't aligned with reality. He'd also been having periods of calm where he was capable of conversing and expressing his emotions. What he was asking for hadn't changed: to be listened to, treated with care and to have his say in things.

I can clearly remember the times Ferid tried to speak with the hospital staff. I can picture him waiting to catch his psychiatrist's attention as the man was leaving the room and, when he didn't, politely calling him over. But his sentence vanished into thin air as he saw the imposing doctor wave his hand dismissively and call over to me, "Tell your son to take his meds!"

I thought to myself, "You must have lost it too, because you're the only one who understands Ferid. Your unconditional love as a mother must mean you can't be objective. You can't see the signs the way they can. They know best." It was a thought that frightened me, and I decided to trust the doctors and follow their lead—after all, they'd studied cases like my son's and worked with similar patients. I choked back questions I knew would earn answers that were evasive, incomplete or flat-out wrong. My judgement was skewed by so many factors: fear, guilt, insufficient knowledge, exhaustion, pressure… the list goes on.

When you hear "schizophrenia," what usually comes to mind is that it's one of the most unliviable and stigmatized of illnesses. Bearing the weight of this forces you to accept almost anything, just so you can make it through. "Schizophrenia" is one of the most violent words I know. Today even the word "crazy" sounds gentler to our ears.

"Free and enlightened" consent

Article 10 of the *Civil Code of Québec* states "Every person is inviolable and is entitled to the integrity of his person. Except in cases provided for by law, no one may interfere with his person without his free and enlightened consent."[1] In this context, "free" means that consent must not be subject to constraints and "enlightened" means that there must be full knowledge of the facts, after the person has received all the relevant information.[2] In terms of mental health, this means that no one can coerce you into treatment—for example, by uttering threats.[3] You also have the right to ask any and all questions related to your diagnosis and the results from the assessments you've undergone, about the recommended treatments and their risks and side effects, and about alternative therapy methods if you don't agree to medication. This is all spelled out in the legislation. The issue lies in determining whether the patient's mental state compromises their ability to give consent. If a healthcare facility or physician deems the person unable to give consent, they must prove it before the Quebec Superior Court. Lawyers enter the picture if the psychiatrist encounters resistance from the patient; when this occurs it is generally done very quickly after hospitalization. It's no wonder people diagnosed with mental disorders feel that care suddenly shifts from being looked after to being locked up.

If the patient is deemed unable to consent, a person authorized by law or mandated by the court can make decisions in their place. Article 12 of the *Civil Code* specifies, however, that the representative must, inasmuch as possible, respect the patient's wishes (even if these wishes are contrary to their own). The patient can therefore maintain refusal of treatment if they wish.

The representative's consent must also be free and enlightened. This means if they need to address the court to make decisions for the patient, they must be informed of all relevant details, particularly the nature of the treatments and their benefits, risks and side effects, since decisions for the patient can have serious effects.

A disregard for protocol

Since it had been established that Ferid, who had been calling himself Jesus, was unable to consent to care, it fell to us to authorize the hospital to file a request with the Superior Court. We finally agreed, but it was over the phone, under pressure and out of desperation. Was our consent "free and enlightened"? What information had they given us? And what about the formal diagnosis? We didn't understand the condition's complexity. We weren't aware of treatment options or how long they'd last, or what their benefits or risks were. None of the staff on the team working with Ferid had felt it necessary to explain the nature of any external resources, such as transition groups and day centres. And yet the team was well aware of Ferid's hesitations when it came to the day program.

Unfortunately, we're not the only ones to have had this experience, it seems. The testimony of so many organizations and the complaints that have been filed indicate clearly that while commendable and reassuring in theory, the guidelines set out in the *Civil Code* are not always respected or adhered to. The Quebec association of intervention groups advocating for mental health rights (AGIDD-SMQ) has even carried out an investigation that reveals just how powerless we are in the wake of court decisions.[4]

According to the AGIDD-SMQ study, the courts are obligated to adhere to the psychiatrists' decisions, since judges do not possess the expertise required to adapt prescriptions and treatment authorizations to the specific cases of people with mental disorders. The AGIDD-SMQ believes that a court order for treatment must remain a "measure of exception since it infringes

Quebec's *Charter of Human Rights and Freedoms* and the *Canadian Charter of Rights and Freedoms* in terms of inviolability of the person and their right to integrity."[5] The authorisation is granted for a period of two, three or even five years, without any possibility of review.

> Generally, people face this court procedure uninformed, without the chance to address the judge and without a lawyer. The fact that it is impossible to review decisions is particularly tragic, since a person's situation can change over such a long period of time and because psychiatric medications and other intrusive treatments have a wide range of effects on an individual. [...]
>
> The court order for treatment [is delivered like a] blank cheque to the attending physician. Out of 150 petitions, 149 included a high-dose prescription. They require jointly taking different classes of psychiatric medication [...]. [They] are very poorly detailed, which allows the attending physician to try one or more treatments and make modifications without the person's consent.[6]

We should have been able to ask questions about the drugs he was prescribed. We should have been able to ask for individualized treatment based on a personal recovery plan, which is common practice at most other hospital centres. We should have been able to ask them to listen to Ferid and to demand that he be transferred to the hospital of his choosing. But we just had no idea.

21. Meeting the Social Worker, or Autoposy of an Act of Sabotage

Ferid's hospital treatment team included a social worker who was supposed to have begun working with him as of his first hospitalization in 2009. Given the recovery program's top-down approach and Ferid's categorical refusal to adhere to it, she'd had nothing to propose. In or outside hospital walls. This being the case, she could in no way claim to know my son.

It's March 2013 and this same social worker is in charge of Ferid's case during his second hospital stay. As our meeting with her and the resident doctor is about to begin, she confidentally and theatrically declares in the hallway that she "knows Ferid well!" This is a fairly inappropriate way to begin things with a family who has never had contact with her. She strongly recommends that we place Ferid in a supervised apartment. We have no idea how this kind of housing situation works.

"You're not doing him any favours by keeping him at home," she says. "He needs to learn to be independent. He can't keep clinging to your apron strings forever."

I admit that she has a point. But we don't want to send Ferid just anywhere. We voice our concerns and ask her to help us find somewhere that's a good fit. She doesn't exactly go out of her way to provide us information, but promises, at least, to "work on it." Usually social workers have relevant literature to give the parents. They sometimes even come along on visits to potential housing. My daughter naively floats a different idea: what if we sold our two apartments to buy a big family home where we can all live together and help each other? The idea is so full of love; it shows just how much she wants to support her brother. But our social worker doesn't believe it would help Ferid to be more independent, that he won't have anyone to socialize with. Our thought is, "Don't we count?" I ask her about the group home clientele. At this point I don't know the difference between supervised housing and group homes, and even less so who lives in them. She evades my question with empty chatter instead of providing us the tools to make an informed decision. Our faces fall. My daughter is on the verge of tears. Furious and distraught, she goes to find the kind and attentive young resident doctor. We feel lucky to have met a charitable soul who understands our struggles and discreetly validates our outrage.

"What do you think about placing Ferid in a supervised environment? Is there a chance he could be a victim of violence or abuse there?"

"Yes. It's a mixed group. There are often people with addiction issues who can be violent," she tells Jasmina.

We're at a crossroads, weighing the need to offer Ferid a challenge against our fear of exposing him to a potentially stressful or dangerous situation. I'd spent several long years building trust with my son and I wasn't ready to risk losing that for a sense of independence. It certainly wasn't worth redescending into hell for the umpteenth time. But we let ourselves be convinced otherwise. We asked the social worker to set up visits so we could tour different locations before we made a decision. One week later, we reconvene as planned. Once again, the social worker doesn't wait until we're in private but, right in the hallway, exclaims, "Oh, what a shame! There was a free room right near the hospital that was just given to someone else."

My daughter is taken aback. "What? We told you we were looking! And you were supposed to help us find options! Why are you telling us now?"

"Oh, it's a long process... It's not that simple. You don't just snap your fingers! You have to take the steps yourself, contact the CLSC..."

We're stunned. We're at a loss for words. Everything we'd agreed to during our first meeting with this woman now appears to have been thrown out the window. She seems to have decided it's no longer her job to find the patient a spot in supervised accommodation; it's ours! And once we're all sitting down, she starts tapping her foot impatiently, checking her watch and staring at the ceiling. We're off to a bad start. During the meeting, the resident doctor in psychiatry tells us about Ferid's progress, his strengths and his needs. She's attentive, composed and present. Ferid will be discharged in a week and my daughter gets straight to the point.

"We're here as his family. And the doctor is here as his psychiatrist and is doing her job. And how about you? Why are you here?"

The social worker doesn't answer. She searches for something to say, while we reiterate the terms of the agreement established during our previous meeting.

"You clearly advised us to place my brother into supervised housing. You convinced us it was the right decision and we agreed that you would start looking at possible placements. Now you've come to this meeting with nothing to propose."

The social worker stands up. "In any case, we can't decide for Ferid. We need to ask him what he thinks!" she shoots back at us.

She's combative at every turn, and she's shamefully using my son as fodder. She asks Ferid, who's waiting outside, to come into the room. He is just as clueless as we'd been about supervised housing.

"So," she starts authoritatively, "how do you feel about going to live in a group home? You'll have to be independent and look after yourself. You'll live with other people and mom won't be there to

cook all your meals and do everything for you..."
Her every sentence is rife with condescendance,
scorn and arrogance. She takes us by surprise and
flips things on us: all of a sudden my daughter and
I are the ones who want to wash our hands of Ferid
without a second thought. It's a warped situation—
and it's destructive. Startled, Ferid looks around
the room to try to understand what's going on.
He has just joined the conversation, so he doesn't
understand what she's referring to. She briefly
explains.

"And the rent for the room is $850 per month!
Can you afford it?" She sets out this staggering
sum to scare him, and she hits her mark. That's
his entire disability cheque.

"But there won't be anything left after the
rent," answers Ferid.

"Well, that's why it's best for you to live with
your mom. You'll have everything you need and
you won't need to pay, and she'll be able to keep
looking after you!"

The social worker speaks to my son with disdain and disrespect, not as an adult but as a child
who is incapable of making a judgmental call,
manipulating him emotionally and exploiting
his weaknesses to lead him where she wants him.
My daughter and I are aghast. She has positioned
us as Ferid's enemy and persecutors; she is his
saviour. She throws all three of us into a state of
confusion and drives us completely off course.
She has sabotaged the meeting with a few cutting

sentences and comes out the winner. We need to minimize the damage and, above all, reassure Ferid. We decide that the best solution is for him to continue living with us. This is the only interaction we have with this woman concerning Ferid.

We file a complaint with the Ombudsman's office regarding the social worker's lack of professionalism. They give us an answer that skirts around her behaviour and focuses on facts with no bearing on the issue. In addition to faulty explanations, they paint a skewed portrait of Ferid and his actions to justify her behaviour.

The cumulative effect of administrative roadblocks and insufficient support from the treatment team heightened our feeling of helplessness in the face of Ferid's mental illness and solidified our distrust of hospitals—the psychiatrist who doesn't stop in the hallway to answer a despairing mother and her son searching for reassurance, a resident doctor who brutally tells Jasmina, "Your brother will probably never marry or have children or live a full life," the deliberate silence of the medical staff... it all drains hope. The dysfunctional health system, deaf to cries of suffering, is responsible for a second mental disorder: all the members of our family—my children, their father and I—lived through this period in a state of extreme anxiety and with an almost continual feeling of despair. This kind of distress can't be written off as a chemical imbalance.

Hope: cornerstone to recovery

The key factor in recovery is undoubtedly hope. But reviving hope in people living with psychotic disorders takes concerted effort. Here's what psychiatrist Marie-Luce Quintal said in 2011 during an interview with Marie-Laurence Poirel, a professor at the Université de Montréal's School of Social Work.

> **MLQ**: I feel like we've gone backwards. We were more focused on rehabilitation 10 years ago. Right now I find we invest less in that clientele—the severely psychotic. And there's too much staff turnover [...] I find that there's not really a goal in sight. We're not going to get anywhere hiring people who don't know much about mental illness. [...] It's going to take people who are familiar with it, who know what these people need, who know what rehabilitation is, who know what recovery is and who want to put the effort in. [...] We can't improvise when it comes to our most vulnerable clientele.
>
> **MLP**: How has having a peer support worker changed things?
>
> **MLQ**: In a few ways. First in terms of giving the users hope. Our clientele have severe psychotic disorders, as well as adjustment disorders—they're often drug-resistant. Meeting someone who tells you they had a psychotic disorder and made it through, that they have a job now—it gives a kind of a hope that we can't offer. And it reminds us as professionals what we're doing is important, that people can get through it.

MLP: Can you tell me a bit about how you work with the people you're treating?

MLQ: Most of what we do is based on an intervention plan. It's a plan that has been modified so it can be self-managed. The person makes their own plan, giving them the power to act. First off the person uses the short guide we've developed and establishes a plan for the future. And that's non-negotable; we never try to alter this goal. After that we work with them. If someone says "I want to be the prime minister," we could say "Maybe we can start by finishing high school or studying politics." We do this in steps, but we don't try to change a person's life plan. Then they examine their strengths. We try to approach things based on the person's strength's in all aspects of recovery. So the person looks at all their strengths and then chooses the ones they want to work with. And the same goes for difficultes—the person chooses three difficulties they want to work on.[1]

Suzanne Lamarre, psychiatrist and professor at McGill University's Department of Psychiatry, worked in emergency psychiatry for numerous years and notes the following:

Affording very little importance to a person's autonomy (i.e., their crucial involvement in the success of therapeutic interventions aimed at making them independent citizens) is a fundamental error that diverts caregivers from their treatment goals, often after services are restructured or methods changed. Priority is often afforded instead to diagnosis and treatment.[2]

Dr. Lamarre raises the point that the "moral treatment" approach promoted by pioneering psychiatrist Philippe Pinel in his *Treatise on Insanity* (original French title: *Traité médico-philosophique de l'aliénation mentale, ou la manie*) published in 1801 "was founded on a humanist and scientific approach. Pinel believed there is always a healthy part of a person living with mental illness and that by addressing this healthy side, we should be able to make the symptoms that alientated the individual in question disappear."[3]

I can still picture my son watching the medical staff walk by, hoping someone will listen. In vain. Though there isn't time alloted for this type of care, it can make all the difference, since creating connections is the best way to start the recovery process. "I know I'm sick and I have to do what the doctors tell me, but I'm also a person and I have a right to be heard," he'd often say to me. And rightly so. He was simply reminding us that the patient is a person, not an illness.

The World Health Organization estimates 450 million people across the globe live with a mental disorder and that, in 2009, depression will be the second largest cause of disability in the world, after cardiovascular diseases. In Canada the Fédération des familles et amis de la personne atteinte de maladie mentale (FFAPAMM, family and friends support network) found that in 2009, 25 to 30 percent of work absenteeism could be attributed to a mental health disorder, resulting in 35 million work days lost. And prejudice is still not a thing of the past: according to the Canadian Medical Association, only 50 percent of Canadians would feel comfortable telling their friends they have a family member with a mental disorder.[4]

Yet here in Canada, we have many youth who hear voices and experience delusions. They are strong, likeable people often with smiles on their faces. Smiles that search for the approval of others to exist, that say "I'm here, I may be from another planet, but I can bring you there if you want to come with me for a while, you'll see, I'm not dangerous. Also your son is really nice. He's doing well, you know..." What does it matter that their ideas are scattered? It's not the veracity of these conversations that is important, it's the extraordinary path these people take to reach us—this should be what moves us and encourages us to accept that we're not always in the same dimension at the same moment.

I wonder what kind of a world we've created, where we exclude those who dream differently, whose journeys happen off the rails. Don't they belong too? Haven't we had nightmares that resemble their realities? Are they that different from us? Why don't they have the right to be different? We need to find ways for the border between our world and theirs to become a space where we can come together and exchange with one another.

22. Other Options

Luckily not all doctors and psychiatric workers can be lumped together. Actively listening to patients is something many medical professionals recommend, in addition to dialogue, mediation with their voices and support in reclaiming personal power. As André Paradis notes, psychiatrists Ronald D. Laing and David Cooper, two other major figures in the antipsychiatry movement, were already proposing something revolutionary in the 1970s—an approach that didn't simply reduce the individual to a spectrum of symptoms:

> They asked medical professionals to leave behind a treatment hierarchy based on a provider-patient model and the safety of labels, to see medication only as a means of respite to facilitate treatment of the essential, and to leave patients the time and space needed to engage in their own healing processes.[1]

The idea of power-sharing means that a health professional works together with the patient and recognizes their expertise. Contrary to a therapeutic relationship based on a paternalistic model between the all-knowing expert and passive patient,[2] a power-sharing relationship balances and returns power to the person trying to recover. It is this focus on recognizing the person's individuality and uniqueness that fuels a patient's desire and hope for recovery. Do we need to break ranks to be heard? It seems like that's the only real way to change things.

American psychologist Carl Rogers believes that a situation's emotional content is more important than the rational facts. To encourage free expression, Rogers developed an active listening approach that involves "using questioning and paraphrasing techniques to clarify the message of one's interlocutor, make sure that one has understood it correctly and provide evidence of this understanding."[3] He points out that it is founded on non-directive techniques and empathy "showing respect and trust towards one's interlocutors, so that they may drop their guard and express themselves as freely as possible." This is the kind of approach that would have greatly benefited Ferid.

Psychiatrist Marie-Luce Quintal states that, "in moments of suffering and incomprehension, people need to make sense of their situation and spirituality often helps, in a larger sense, no matter what religion it happens to be."[4] Dr. Quintal believes it's easy to understand why a person might feel the urge to express religion's importance in their life within the framework of a therapeutic relationship.

What was the right thing to answer Ferid when he told me, amid an episode of psychosis, that he was Christ? As a Muslim, should I have disowned him? Should I have invoked the fury of Allah and begged him to see reason? Or begged him to reconsider? Told him I was ashamed? God did not demand anything beyond my power. According to the Muslim scholar At-Tirmidhī, the messenger of God said, "Have mercy upon those on Earth, so that He who is in Heaven may have mercy upon you." From this, I take away that mercy is for everyone.

Alternative treatment

Ferid loved video games, and he was a whiz at computers. A program based around this kind of technology could have been a good way for him to express himself. Unfortunately, he wasn't the one deciding on his treatment.

If you refuse treatment, instead of subjecting the therapeutic relationship to strict legal procedures—based on laws that are often rigid or downright inapplicable—psychiatry staff should be asking themselves whether the treatment works for that patient's unique reality. The health system still has miles to go in addressing the suffering and needs of most; that's perfectly clear when you hear or read about the experiences of former patients who were lucky enough to make it through to tell the tale. Ferid once recounted how he and other patients had watched staff on the psychiatry ward forcefully hold a patient down in an isolation room and inject him with drugs—trauma on multiple levels.

There are so many alternative resources available. Here are a few:

- The **peer support network** (Réseau des pairs aidants) that brings together people who have recovered from mental health disorders; they support and assist patients on the same road to recovery. More and more mental health institutions are teaming up with peer support workers, as they offer patients an invaluable relationship of trust and a sense of understanding through shared experience.
- **Spiritual care providers** are also invaluable support workers to whom patients and their family can turn, even in the hospital environment. It's a right. Their support and listening are a key part of recovery. There are also various therapies based on listening to religious delusions that allow the individual to work through inner conflict, with a trained spiritual care provider acting as intermediary.
- **Mental health organizations** provide a space to share experiences with others, breaking the isolation and making it easier to live with our problems. Among these organizations there is Prise II, which offers programs based on user interests and goals, and Réseau d'entendeurs

de voix québécois (REVQuébécois), where people who experience psychosis learn how to cope with their voices. REV was founded in 2009 and has 13 centres in Quebec, including 4 in Montreal.

- *La renaissance* is a quarterly newsletter published by **Action Autonomie**, a mental rights advocacy collective in Montreal. It is distributed for free in community organizations and CLSCs. It includes a space devoted to real-life experiences, as well as a legal rights section with vital information about rights most people are unaware of. It's also useful to know that family members of a person living with a mental disorder can receive support from someone at Action Autonomie in certain cases—something I benefited from.

- **Animal-assisted therapy (zootherapy)** has existed in Quebec since 1990. This type of therapy, which is supposedly costly for our health system, is practiced in certain hospital centres, such as the Douglas Mental Health University Institute, the Institut de zoothérapie du Québec (the province's animal-assisted therapy institute) and the Rivière-des-Prairies hospital. According to animal-assisted therapists, the unconditional love animals provide boosts patients' well-being and self-esteem. Petting an animal reduces stress and blood pressure, and encourages conversation. Pet therapy has also been proven to have a positive effect on cancer patients and children with autism.

When he lived alone, Ferid had several cats that he took good care of, despite his limited resources. Later he would also look after his brother's cat and two budgies. It was a calming, rewarding ritual. It was also a topic of conversation and the subject of jokes. One week after he died, the first budgie died. The second bird escaped from its cage several days later.

The hospital environment must not only encourage collaboration with alternative resources, but also act as the bridge between patients, parents, friends and external professionals, so that the service chain remains unbroken.

23. Hope Fraught with Hazard

Ferid is still determined to get better despite all the blunders, disappointments and the tepid therapeutic relationship. He's "180 percent ready to change," he tells the treatment team in a meeting. During the 34-day hospital stay, he's gained some of his strength back but is still fragile. They've prescribed him Abilify, a brand-new antipsychotic. Ferid seems determined to keep taking it, despite the extrapyramidal symptoms (mainly anxiety, which they try treating with another drug).

He'll be discharged soon. He's developed a routine and friendships on the ward, but he'll have to leave that all behind to take the next step. As per hospital protocol, he'll spend two trial days at home first.

The first thing he wants to do on our way home is get a hamburger. We stop at McDonald's. Adam's waiting at home, and Ferid thinks to buy him a meal too. I can breathe easier now that Ferid is no longer inside those sad hospital walls. When I look at him, I feel hopeful.

It's a rocky first night. The next day Ferid isn't feeling well and wants to go back to the ward. He isn't ready to come home. "But how come?" He won't talk to me about it. Maybe he can speak with someone from his treatment team? Along with this not knowing comes mounting guilt. Four days later, Ferid is released from the hospital for good and referred to the day hospital for follow-up. Just looking at him, it's clear how vulnerable he's feeling.

Ferid has always been reserved and proud. It's part of his nature, not the illness. He's living in our basement. He has his own bedroom, kitchenette, bathroom, living room and separate entrance, giving him his freedom and independence. (There are only two bedrooms upstairs: the very small one belongs to Adam and the other one is mine— which Ferid doesn't want.) It's dark downstairs, but he can come up for meals and spend evenings with us.

The week Ferid came home from the hospital is a blur. I can recall only a few details. One thing is certain: on Sunday, April 14, 2013, my son woke up before me and came into my room. He felt depressed, and his entire body hurt. He wanted to go back to the hospital; so we went.

24. April 14, 2013: The Emergency Room

We automatically make our way to the psychiatry department where Ferid was admitted one month earlier, hoping to see a member of his treatment team. But his file has already been closed. The receptionist won't hear us out and sends us back to square one: Emergency. I desperately explain that my son has been a patient here before and is being followed as an outpatient. But she won't budge. Back to square one: the emergency room.

The bureaucracy and absurdly dysfunctional system infuriate me. I hate being in this place, but have no other choice. Fuming, I go up and down never-ending staircases and hallways with Ferid in tow. We do the whole process again from the beginning. We present ourselves at triage, where Ferid once again declines his identity. We both reiterate that Ferid has just been discharged from the hospital. Can't we go directly to psychiatry? Isn't that logical? Are there hospitals that coordinate care in a more intelligent, efficient way?

We spend eight hours in a packed waiting room. Ferid suffers in silence. I suffer too, out of helplessness. He's triaged and a medical student finally sees us. She reads off the endless list of depression symptoms, which we already know by heart. Ferid complies and adds, pointing to the parts of his body that are in pain, "My whole body feels like it's on fire. I can't stand it. I feel so empty." I ask the young woman what she thinks, and she replies that those are symptoms of schizoaffective disorder. Another diagnosis. Apparently even a student doctor can switch out a diagnosis at random with another DSM classification, another label that legitimizes a profession I regard today with a great deal of mistrust. Why not simply admit my son is still recovering and was released too quickly? Why not look at the side effects of Abilify—the new drug with such an evocative name—that Ferid has been prescribed? It seems the logical place to start.

None of the three medical staff who examine Ferid that day ask any questions related to the side effects of his medication. It isn't their problem, I guess? The student slips out of the room. Then it's the resident's turn. Same list of questions, same answers. She leaves. Then the psychiatrist arrives and asks even more questions, before finally coming to the root.

"Are you having suicidal thoughts?"

"Yes."

"Do you have a plan to commit suicide?"

"No."

Ferid tells the psychiatrist he wants to die so that he doesn't have to suffer this way anymore, explaining again that his body hurts all over and he's weighed down by a sense of emptiness. I'm nervous when I hear him say this. I know my son: he has a high threshold for pain and he's not the kind to complain.

"Give me something to make it stop."

The psychiatrist asks if he's taking his medication. Yes, he is. She doesn't go into the possibility of side effects. In any case, we don't know what they are. She leaves and then comes back.

"You need to come to the day hospital tomorrow."

Ferid isn't the kind to insist, so I interrupt her, despairingly:

"Please do something for him, Doctor. He won't go to the day hospital." I could barely contain my frustration. I didn't expect them to send us back home when Ferid is visibly in unbearable pain and asking for help.

"Can't you do something for him now? Please?" I ask the psychiatrist, who looks around the same age as me and likely has children of her own.

"He's suffering."

"There aren't enough symptoms of depression to prescribe him anything." She asks Ferid one last question: "What do you want us to do?"

"To stop the suffering." My son patiently looks at her, hoping for help that no one seems able to offer. I can replay this scene in my head as clearly as if it were yesterday. And it still hurts.

"Go to the day hospital tomorrow."

I feel broken, powerless, empty. Beneath our words is a heavy silence that nothing can lift. Leaving Emergency we're both hurting. I'd fruit-lessly tried to explain that my son had little rea-son to want to show up at the day hospital, that he'd never created meaningful connections with the staff there. But she ignored my pleas, even though I was Ferid's caregiver and the person who knew him best. She just repeated the same advice.

Ferid was quiet the whole way home. The calm made me nervous. Did I bring up the day hos-pital again? That place he'd never liked? I don't remember, but I think I may have.

"You should go, don't you think?"

Ferid nodded. After all, psychiatrists must be better placed to judge our level of suffering and how best to manage it. To decide when and where to relieve it. And sometimes, for Ferid and many others, you have to wait until tomorrow.

My son went only once to the day hospital, where they'd already closed his file. We had to call the person in charge for permission to reopen it so Ferid could be seen on that fateful Monday, April 15, 2013.

25. April 15, 2013

"It is more important to know what sort of person has a disease than to know what sort of disease a person has."
–Hippocrates

The day after we are sent home from Emergency, I call the day hospital's director to try to convince him of Ferid's real, urgent needs and vulnerable state. It doesn't take long for the conversation to take a different track; the man is impatient, irritated, seemingly incapable of active listening. He fixates on Ferid's track record, judging his attitude and feigning incomprehension as to why Ferid took no interest in the activities his team proposed the last time. I try to communicate, but the director's ill humour takes over the conversation, to the point that it feels like reopening Ferid's file would be giving us one final chance.

Assailed from all directions, I attempt to motivate Ferid to get ready to go back to the day hospital. He agrees, then changes his mind at the last minute. I feel hurt, angry and powerless. The whole situation ignites a fuse I can't put out. His refusal triggers the only action I regret. I understand and can imagine all the reasons he doesn't want to go—he's the only one truly able to judge whether it will help. But I don't have the power to help him anymore. I feel trapped, beyond powerless, and try one last time to change his mind. When he resists, I tell him that's it, "From now on, you're on your own if you need to go to the hospital. I won't be there to go with you."

Anger clears a path, destroying everything in its wake. My son watches me from across the room without a word. I feel defeated, helpless, at a loss. And I hate myself for it. This is how the seriously ill get worn down. How suicide becomes a way out. For good.

The link between suicide and schizophrenia

In their book *Comprendre le suicide* (Understanding suicide), Brian Mishara and Michel Tousignant discuss schizophrenia:

> The diagnosis [of schizophrenia] presents an elevated risk of suicide, equal to that of depression and bipolar disorders, i.e., 1 out of 10. [...] The paranoid form of the illness poses a higher risk than other forms, and the risk increases if depression is present. These states [...] represent a danger because the person is no longer able to realize that their quality of life is diminishing.[1]

The DSM-5 notes:

Approximately 5–6 percent of individuals with schizophrenia die by suicide, about 20 percent attempt suicide on one or more occasions, and many more have significant suicidal ideation. Suicidal behavior is sometimes in response to command hallucinations [...]. Other risk factors including having depressive symptoms or feelings of hopelessness [...] and the risk is higher, also, in the period after a psychotic episode or hospital discharge.[2]

Ferid's file should have been in the hospital's computers since September 2009. His family history, hospitalizations, patient information, follow-ups—everything should have been recorded. Some intelligent soul should have considered his profile, including his refusals for follow-up. Ferid was never overly inclined to cooperate, so showing up at Emergency of his own volition was a sign of how much he knew he needed help, and how urgently. His first diagnosis was paranoid schizophrenia. Did they consider the anxiety that must have accompanied his second psychotic episode? Or the medication's side effects? Ferid wasn't a regular at Emergency. He couldn't be accused of abusing the health system or wielding his illness as a weapon. He had a strong threshold for pain. He didn't like the hospital, or its services. But he went out of desperation. He was visibly anguished. But he wasn't able to access the help he needed, when he needed it.

Today, I let my son's story pour out onto the page. I respect his decision not to go to the day hospital, where he didn't feel comfortable. Nobody could know better than he could. I bitterly regret letting my anger take hold, and the words that came out of my mouth without thinking. I loved him through all my pain, helplessness and despair. I wanted him to get better, but I know now that he made the right decision.

The hospital had adopted a hard line with patients with mental disorders and a subordinator-subordinate relationship. There wasn't much space for a sick person's opinion. From the first hospital stay to his last cry for help, Ferid experienced nothing but trauma within those walls. We were shocked by all that was lacking: knowledge, information, time, support, staff, humanism and compassion. What would it have cost the psychiatric staff to suggest alternatives (which I would have paid for myself)? I asked questions. I tried to find answers. I wanted to be involved. I used my best judgement, treated everyone with respect. By September 2009 I had already expressed the need for someone to be with my son during his psychotic episode, to be at his side while he was assailed by voices telling him terrible things. There wasn't a single staff member who thought to tell us about the Hearing Voices Network, for instance?

If the user is the very reason health services exist, as Quebec law states, then as a citizen I ask: what right do hospital staff have to hinder access to external resources? The simple answer is that they're not breaking any laws by remaining silent. It's therefore a question of conscience. But I'm not as naive as I once was. I know that hospitals are reluctant to collaborate with organizations offering alternative non-invasive treatment. Why? Because hospital staff fear the patient will exert their right to refuse drugs in favour of alternative care. And why not, if that's what works?

And as always, it's a question of money. Treatment centred around the patient's needs, that consider a mental disorder's underlying causes, cost more and take longer than writing out a prescription. Often all these pills do is stifle behaviour that society finds problematic. Costs related to patient care aren't the only thing at stake: when someone suffers, their family takes the collateral damage, as quality of life plummets and exhaustion sets in. Especially if the caregiver is, as I was, the only family support person. Mental health disorders create a home life that's often heavy and disheartening, weighing on the family for what can be years.

What about patients with other illnesses? Do they have recourse to support systems beyond medication, such as a priest, psychologist or peer support worker? Do they encounter the same closed-mindedness from staff? In treating mental health disorders, peer support is a precious resource that can complement the knowledge of the medical staff, since it starts where their expertise leaves off. Peer support workers have travelled the long road to recovery and understand what it is like to experience psychosis. They are well versed in pain, but also hope. There is a Moroccan proverb that says, "Seek advice from the ill, not the doctor." Like all disciplines, medicine has its limitations, shortcomings and dangers.

26. Life After Ferid

There is no question that grief marks the start of a new life. At first, it is an open wound that takes all physical and mental energy, and requires strategies, escapes and roundabout methods to patch. That others have lived through the same offers solace, and life forces us to snap back to the present, amid tears and anxious laughter. But the pain never really goes away. We just learn how to live with it.

I first came across Action Autonomie online. As I mentioned before, the organization supports people with mental health disorders and their loved ones, advocating for mental health rights. This is how I met Kevin, my guardian angel. His empathy and willingness to listen have been invaluable.

The first thing Kevin recommended was for me to contact the coroner to request an investigation into the exact circumstances of my son's death. I was initially reticent at the idea of having the body exhumed, but I agreed to call. My conversation with the coroner unfortunately unfolded like all my other failed attempts at being heard as the parent of someone with a mental disorder.

"I've consulted your son's medical file, Mrs. Ferkovic. He should have taken his medication," he promptly said, implying this was *all Ferid had to do*. "Medication has saved a lot of lives over the past few years."

"But the problem," I tried, futilely, to explain, "is that my son went to Emergency for help because he was in pain, and he was sent home..."

"Right, well, you'll need to file a complaint with the hospital."

I'm an emotional person who gets flustered when I come up against resistance. It didn't occur to me to calmly reply that my son was medicated when he was sent home from the hospital, but that he had returned because he was in pain and having suicidal thoughts, and that the decision of the emergency-room psychiatrist was not what we had expected. Crestfallen and searching for answers, I'd wanted to turn to someone independent of the hospital that had failed my son—a place I'd completely lost trust in. And here I was, once again feeling caught in a system that was sending me right back to square one.

The coroner hastily delivered his unequivocal opinion: Ferid was the sole person responsible for what had happened to him. In his eyes Ferid remained the uncooperative patient of 2009. Ferid's medical file, which we had never been granted access to, said it all. The stack of notes protected by the *Privacy Act* was working against him. Did it also detail the unnecessary pain Zyprexa had caused him? This antipsychotic has had, after all, class actions filed and criminal fines levied against it well before Ferid's first hospital stay, both in Canada and the U.S. Did it portray an intelligent young man fully able to decide how he wanted to spend his time? Was there anything in that file, accessible only to the staff, that reflected the person my son actually was?

His medical file appeared to list the series of coercive interventions he'd received, treatment based on a mechanical and dehumanizing framework; it seemed limited to cold facts that painted a portrait of an uncooperative psychiatric patient who was disliked and out of institutional control.

If my son had known half of what I know today, particularly that he had the right to refuse all medication and demand alternative treatment without fear of legal reprisals, likely I wouldn't be here today guilt-ridden, stuck in a never-ending process. The indifference, cruelty, silence and lack of accountability are as lethal as bombs being hurled through a clear sky. These deaths represent the failures of a system that is sick and knows it. If you need proof, take a look at the people sleeping on the streets of our city on freezing winter nights. We're supposed to believe that's a choice?

Speaking to the coroner made me realize that I wouldn't find any allies within the medical system. I had to look elsewhere.

The link between prescription drugs and suicide

Despite the *omertà* that prevails in the drug industry and related sectors, more and more people are coming forward with their stories. These are people who have lost a child, a brother, a spouse because of antidepressants, psychiatric drugs or other psychostimulants and their accounts are now omnipresent online. Their stories counter a dangerous culture of silence and collusion among pharmaceutical giants, governmental authorities and even certain organizations that claim to advocate for people with mental disorders.

In his book on pharmaceutical industry corruption, Peter C. Gøtzsche denounces the repeated acts of fraud in the drug industry, particularly manipulation of data and lies propagated about the safety and effectiveness of the popular antidepressant Paxil.[1] Study 329 funded by GlaxoSmithKline (GSK), Paxil's manufacturer, concluded that the antidepressant was "generally well tolerated and effective for major depression in adolescents [and children]," while the company had internal documents proving the contrary.[2] In the United States, this antidepressant was prescribed to children and teens on more than two million occasions. In 2004, New York's attorney general sued GlaxoSmithKline for "repeated and persistent fraud."[3] In 2012, GSK pleaded guilty and paid a record $3 billion for the unlawful promotion of paroxetine (Paxil) and additional drugs.[4]

Gøtzsche also speaks about "concealing suicides and suicide attempts in clinical trials."[5] It's not only scientists on drug company payrolls engaging in fraud; the problem goes all the way to the top of the Food and Drug Administration (FDA).

> FDA reviewers and independent researchers found that the big companies had concealed cases of suicidal thoughts and acts by labelling them "emotional lability." However, the FDA bosses suppressed this information. When safety officer Andrew Mosholder concluded that SSRIs [Selective Serotonin Reuptake Inhibitors] cause increased suicidality among teenagers, the FDA prevented him from presenting his findings at an advisory meeting and suppressed his report. When the report was leaked, the FDA's reaction was to do a criminal investigation into the leak.[6]

Along the same thinking as Terence Young in *Death by Prescription*, Gøtzsche estimates the following.

> "[A]round 100,000 people die each year in the United States because of the drugs they have taken, even though they take them correctly. Another 100,000 die because of errors, such as too high dose or use of a drug despite contraindications [...]
>
> The European Commission has estimated that adverse reactions kill about 200,000 EU citizens annually. [...] In 2010, heart disease killed

600,000 Americans, cancer 575,000 and chronic lower respiratory disease came third with 140,000 deaths. This means that in the United States and Europe: drugs are the third leading cause of death after heart disease and cancer."[7]

The documentary *Morts sur ordonnance*[8] by Olivier Pighetti focuses on lives lost to the devastating effects of prescription drugs. Dr. Philippe Even is one of the main interviewees of the movie and one of the few specialists to have ardently sounded the alarm about drug risks. He explains that for many people, anxiolytics (anti-anxiety medication) and sleep aids are more addictive than heroine—which is why treatment with these drugs should never extend beyond a few weeks. Dr. Even also notes that for antidepressants that take effect only after two or three weeks, there is a risk of murder and suicide in the first days of taking the drug, after an increase in dose or when stopping medication. British psychiatrist Dr. David Healy corroborates the information. Known for his critical take on the drug industry's role in "marketing" diseases, Healy estimates that 1 in 20 people experience this type of extreme reaction.

On February 24, 2010, Dr. Peter R. Breggin spoke before the U.S. House Committee on Veterans' Affairs and summarized the situation eloquently.[9] His research examines suicidality, suicide attempts and other violent acts caused by antidepressants, and he believes causality between taking these drugs and suicidal behaviour has been scientifically proven. A quote on the cover of his book *Medication Madness* reads "There are hundreds of millions of psychiatric drug prescriptions written annually. Are they doing more harm than good?"[10]

The lure of profit is the leitmotif of these predatory drug companies. Without the integrity of scientists and industry professionals who are fighting to end the slaughter, we all risk being struck down by tragedy at some point in our lives, and left wondering why.

27. Fighting Fatalism

"An advertising budget of $2.4 billion per year spent on Abilify and Seroquel has catapulted these two very so-so and not-so-safe drugs to fifth and sixth place as revenue producers among all of the many medicines sold in America."
–Dr. Allen Frances, *Saving Normal*[1]

Ferid had always been a calm, thoughtful young man. After his second hospitalization, he'd realized he needed help. Instead of circling back to denial or turning inward, he'd decided to take the medication prescribed and expressed a desire to actively participate in the recovery process before even leaving the hospital in April 2013. At that point, he was not exhibiting delusions. His last episode had made a few things clear, and had even brought us closer together.

I can still hear him asking us to find him a private institution. He believed there would be more personalized, higher quality services if we were paying for them. "I have money," he told us. He'd managed to put savings aside even on his meager disability income—since that is what his illness was considered, a "disability." I can picture him after he was released from the hospital, his peaceful expression, shining with hope for the future.

Yet his episode on April 14, 2013 had struck without warning: pain and a burning sensation throughout his entire body, a feeling of emptiness, suicidal thoughts. What could have triggered the break? At the time I never even considered that he was likely suffering from side effects of his new medication.

Abilify: a long list of side effects

On Wikipedia I learn that aripiprazole, marketed under the brand name Abilify, is the sixth atypical antipsychotic to be introduced. It is used to treat schizophrenia, acute mania and mixed bipolar episodes. At first glance, the list of side effects beats all records! In December 2011, Heath Canada approved its use for children 15 and over in the treatment of schizophrenia. And the Société Québécoise de la Schizophrénie rejoiced at the news!

Side effects are possible with any medication, drug, alcohol or chemical substance. When a psychiatrist or general practitioner prescribes a drug, they must inform the patient of all the risks, even minor ones. Let us not forget: it is our right.

When it comes to Abilify, the first of the "precautions" is monitoring hematological parameters to survey changes in blood sugar and cholesterol levels to prevent type 2 diabetes. It can also cause tardive dyskinesia, which involves abnormal, involuntary movement of the tongue, jaw, torso or extremities; this side effect gives rise to other debilitating consequences like social exclusion, isolation and diminished self-esteem and self-worth of the patient. Numerous cases of neuroleptic malignant syndrome, characterized by intense muscular rigidity and fever, have also been reported. Abilify may cause other side effects related to the nervous system including agitation, anxiety, insomnia, dizziness, akathisia (restlessness), extrapyramidal syndrome (types of involuntary movement with neurological basis), trembling, an increase in saliva production, confusion and gait disturbance, difficulty concentrating, dystonia, motor impairment and vasodilatation. In terms of psychiatric side effects, the drug can cause depression as well as manic, schizophrenic or paranoid reactions, hallucinations, hostility, suicidal thoughts, delusions and strange dreams.

In short, Abilify causes side effects worse than those associated with my son's disorder, for which the drug was prescribed! Important note: alongside Zyprexa, Risperdal, Paxil, Trileptal, Seroquel and many other neuroleptics, Abilify is on the long list of drugs that have been subject to lawsuits; it's creator, Bristol-Myers Squibb, was fined US$515 million for off-label promotion in 2007[2] and agreed to pay a $19.5 million settlement in December 2016.[3]

Ferid had been taking Abilify for a month. He felt depressed and suffered from physical burning sensations and thoughts of suicide. He'd explicitly told the psychiatrist this when he was seen at Emergency on April 14, 2013. All she had been concerned with finding out was whether he was taking his medication, without even considering that the drug itself might be the culprit. She simply evaluated whether he was dangerous to himself or others, based on whether he had a plan to kill himself, but didn't assess any other risk factors. She imposed her decision on Ferid, who didn't contest it out of respect for her authority. Few of us feel comfortable contesting medical authority. In the end, my son just gave up.

28. Filing a Complaint: The Long Wait

On April 29, 2013, I email a complaint to the Jewish General Hospital's Commissioner of Complaints and Quality of Service requesting an investigation into how Ferid was treated at Emergency on April 14, 2013. The confirmation of receipt says I'll receive a reply within 45 days, as provided by law.

September arrives and with it another letter. The complaints office gives their sincere apologies for the delay, explaining that the medical examiner currently has a heavy case load. From that point on, I'm like a frog in a pot of water that must acclimate to new temperatures as the heat is slowly turned up to reach boiling point, without making a sound. I don't have the strength to go any further.

My son has left this world, and it is unbearable to think about his suicide. What could push a person who, though suffering, was full of life and the will to live, to commit suicide six days after their release from the hospital? It's true that certain symptoms of schizophrenia, such as aggressive auditory hallucinations, can encourage a person to end their life. But the statistics found online about the unusually high suicide rates among people with schizophrenia rarely account for the following:

- The context surrounding the patient and their loved ones' lived experiences
- The major role of emergency hospital services
- The devastating side effects of prescription drugs
- The health system's serious shortcomings when handling people with mental disorders at all levels of care

In her annual 2014–2015 report, the Quebec Ombudsperson, Raymonde Saint-Germain, laments the situation in a section about mental health: "Are mental health care and services truly a priority for the Ministère de la Santé et des Services Sociaux? Unfortunately, no."[1]

She notes that the need for these services is both crucial and increasing, and that progress on mental health-related cases remains rare. She argues that the health and social services minister should make public the ministry's goals in applying the Act respecting the protection of persons whose mental state presents a danger to themselves or to others, which guides procedure for institutional confinement; these directives were held up for over five years and finally made public in late 2018.[2]

Every death by suicide is unique, just like every life. No one should tell a grieving loved one that many people with schizophrenia and other mental disorders commit suicide—it is flat out insulting—but this is what came out of the mouth of our son's resident psychiatric doctor in 2013. Unfortunately, this kind of attitude is not uncommon.

Hope and happiness

Schizophrenia is often demonized, yet apart from the psychotic episodes, which are indeed traumatic, a person living with the illness can go through remission periods where hope and happiness are not out of reach—assuming they are not placed under pressure and receive adequate medical care, along with community support.

Following Ferid's first hospitalization in 2009, we believed he had lost his spark for life. Something fundamental had broken inside him. He'd become indifferent, distant and detached, without any personal projects on the horizon. We couldn't understand it. We knew so little about the illness, and it was frightening to see how it seemed to have crushed his spirit. At the time his zombie state had been attributed to emotional indifference, a symptom of the schizophrenia. But this pseudo-symptom had only shown up after he began taking Zyprexa.

We continued to believe all blame rested on his illness, likely because of how disempowered we felt due to a lack of information, our exclusion from the recovery process and the treatment team's overwhelming power. But it simply was not the case. Illness is the human body's complex natural response to an underlying problem. Today's medical approach fails to consider the emotional ties and attachments to people and places expressed by patients and their families. In fact, it does not consider much. Patients are seen as simply biological matter that must be treated sporadically, in a vacuum and according to the protocols of a soulless health system.

Open Dialogue therapy, detailed in Chapter 13, encourages a different approach. The patient participates in the recovery process, and solutions are sparked through consensus between the patient, their family members and the treatment team. The patient therefore has power over the outcome.

In his documentary *Take These Broken Wings*,[3] Daniel Mackler—who travelled all the way to Lapland to interview the Open Dialogue team—tells the stories of different individuals, including Catherine Penney and Joanne Greenberg,[4] two women who were diagnosed with schizophrenia at a young age and completely recovered without medication. Their perspectives on the illness and recovery are illuminating. Greenberg speaks about schizophrenia as a complex system of defence mechanisms and protection against the successive abuse and trauma she experienced in her life.

In the documentary numerous experts affirm the need to prioritize compassionate care over all other forms of treatment, especially medication. Dr. Peter Breggin notes:

> The key to helping people, the most fundamental thing, is to help them get over feeling helpless. To help them understand they can actually figure things out and make decisions, make choices. And you can't do that if you're giving medication because you're saying to them, "You can't do it. You need a drug."

In addition to talking about the limitations and dangers of medication and denouncing the drug industry's influence in the healthcare sector, the documentary deconstructs the misinformation and prejudice circulated in our society. We still have not learned to dig deeper when it comes to today's psychiatric practices. A better understanding of the issues would push us to stay proactive and make better choices for ourselves, the people we love and our community as a whole.

29. Duty to Rescue

I received the medical examiner's reply in April 2016, three years after filing my complaint. Coincidentally, it arrived on the deadline to file an official complaint in the courts.[1] It is impossible not to see the connection. I wouldn't be able to seek justice from anyone. In any case I wasn't interested in embarking on a long and costly court proceeding against a system stronger than me, nor was I looking for an amicable agreement that would brush things under the rug. I just wanted them to know what my son had really gone through.

Here is an excerpt from the medical examiner's letter: "On April 14 [2013], Mr. Ferkovic returned to Emergency. His primary complaints were a feeling of emptiness and that he missed the social connections he'd developed after being admitted to the psychiatry unit." First thing: it's stunning how an emergency situation can be reduced to this. My son had not come to the hospital because of a feeling of emptiness or because he was missing his social connections. The letter continues:

After evaluation [...] the doctor judged that your son was depressed due to a change in routine and social isolation. She found no indication that he was a risk to himself or to others. She confirmed that he was taking his medication regularly. She believed that the best course of action was for him to return home and receive follow-up treatment at the day psychiatry hospital. He was advised to return to the hospital if he had suicidal thoughts or a suicide plan.

From my perspective, the two main causes for Ferid's visit to Emergency that day had been carefully omitted from the reply: extreme anguish (manifested in physical pain) and suicidal thoughts. Once these have been lifted from the conversation, there's suddenly nothing to suggest he needed help. The exchange between the psychiatrist and Ferid on that fatal day in April 2013 is still etched into my memory:

"Have you been having suicidal thoughts?"

"Yes."

"Do you have a plan for ending your life?"

"No."

"What would you like us to do?"

"To make the pain stop. I can't go on like this..."

The doctor denied the presence of suicidal thoughts in the medical examiner's inquiry, claiming that she'd suggested Ferid return to Emergency if he had suicidal thoughts or a plan—but she made no such recommendation! She simply advised him to go to the day hospital, even though I'd explained that my son wouldn't go. I'd begged her to help him, because I was sure that an immediate compassionate response would have made him feel secure and calm then and there. But her opinion overruled mine. At the time I felt broken. As caregivers, parents are the ultimate experts. They have knowledge about the patient that psychiatrists and doctors don't possess. Many health professionals recognize this expertise and use it to maximize the patient's chances for recovery.

Here is another excerpt from the medical examiner's reply that illustrates how the situation was turned on its head in favour of the psychiatrist:

> When he left the hospital on April 8 and while he was at Emergency, your son was capable of making decisions. He demonstrated an understanding of his illness. He was aware of the treatment recommended to him and he approved it. Unfortunately he experienced a lapse in judgement. He chose not to follow the recommended treatment.

Response: when my son went to Emergency for help soon after his release from the hospital, his judgement was spot on. He knew he needed immediate help. Answering his call for help should not have been put off to the next day. Ferid did not know the cause of his suffering. He was unaware of the possible side effects of his medication. To reiterate: none of the staff who saw him that evening considered he might be experiencing side effects. I can attest to that. How could the psychiatrist conclude that Ferid had understood and agreed to the proposed treatment if she hadn't even discussed it with him? Sending someone who is highly vulnerable away after a five-minute discussion is not professional care.[2] The psychiatrist made the wrong call. The reply rife with contradictions that she sent to the medical examiner fails to justify her actions.

I contacted Kevin from Action Autonomie because I wanted to write a request for review. This time my request would contain only the facts. I wanted to take a magnifying glass to each element of the medical examiner's answer before submitting it to the review committee. Kevin helped me compose my reply over the course of several meetings.

At home everyone was upset for me. They tried to tell me it was normal that the hospital's response found no fault in the health professional's decision, that it was naive to think I'd get anything more from them. I knew they were right. I hadn't expected an admission of guilt.

Meeting with the review committee

Kevin and I were greeted by three staff members from the Montreal Jewish General Hospital on September 27, 2016. I should note that the review committee had demanded to see my application two weeks prior to our meeting. This gave the members the necessary time to prepare; I did not have the same luxury, since I'd never seen my son's medical file nor did I receive any support whatsoever from the hospital.

It was the first time I'd set foot in the hospital since my son had died. I had the painful feeling of returning to a surreal past. The memories were floating around, ready to overwhelm me, but I kept an emotional distance that let me focus on the task at hand. This mental work took up so much space that I could barely think. As Nelson Mandela once said, "Like a marathon, the last kilometer is the hardest."

In my eyes Ferid had become a silent spokesperson. I wanted people to know he had a loving mother who had cared about him and a loving family who would always remember him. Arriving at our meeting, Kevin and I felt the wind in our faces as the first yellow leaves of the year floated by in the warm light. Is this what resistance looks like? "It doesn't matter," encouraged Kevin with his wide smile. "It's not the result that matters, Sadia, it's the process. It's there, in the steps." I had hoped for more. I wanted things to be different for the people who would cry for help in the ERs of our hospitals after me—so many thoughts to try to console myself. Could Kevin read my mind? He told me again that he was there for me. When a stone is thrown into the water, it creates a ripple. All of this would not be in vain.

I'd pictured walking into some sort of giant oval office and facing a panel of professionals waiting to rip me apart; instead it was three women—two psychiatrists—who courteously ushered us into a small office. They told us their mandate (to hear what I had to say and submit my complaint before the committee) and then listened attentively while I read my complaint, which centered on how the medical examiner's version of the encounter was not, in fact, the reality. The psychiatrists looked surprised.

"Were you in the ER with your son?"

"Yes, I came with him."

And then the question I'd been expecting: "What would you have liked them to do differently that day?"

Kevin had warned me they'd ask me this. He'd advised me not to answer—I wasn't a doctor after all. I replied carefully, hoping they would read between the lines.

"Emergency is emergency. A day centre is a day centre."

I was so close to replying that my son should have been kept in observation that night and seen his physician the next day. That it was a precaution they should have taken given his mental state.

The meeting was brief, but we walked out happy. Kevin and I had carefully prepared our arguments to contest the medical examiner's report, which Kevin had deemed violent, and speak as citizens concerned about the treatment of people with mental disorders. From there the review committee could decide to:

- Ratify the medical examiner's conclusions
- Demand that the medical examiner continue the investigation
- Send a copy of my complaint to the relevant authorities for disciplinary action
- Suggest measures to resolve the matter between the parties.

What was I hoping to get out of the process? First and foremost: to shatter the silence. My complaint could be filed away or destroyed, I had no power over that, but it's impossible to erase the memory of a mother relating the last moments of her son's life and the magnitude of this loss for his family.

In the end the review committee concluded that "the examiner of my complaint [had been] diligent and fair in studying my complaint"—it had taken them three years to write me a letter full of inconsistencies and they had never asked for my version of events. Case closed. But how can a fair decision be rendered if the complainant was never even contacted? When these kinds of aberrations occur it makes you want to question your own sanity.

What would have happened to my son if they'd have kept him in the hospital that night? Would he have found hope again and confidence in himself and others? Would he have decided life was still worth living, despite the stigma, the long road ahead and the faulty system? I believe so.

30. Ferid Ferkovic's Story

I slowly began to realize the full magnitude of the problem I was trying to tackle. I was not the first mother to be devastated by the loss of a child. Far from it. Thousands of other families, in Quebec and beyond, have known, or will sadly one day know, what it is like. A good number of them grieve this loss alone, racked with guilt and grappling to understand.

The subject of suicide remains taboo. It is one of many issues surrounding the fate of people living with mental disorders in our society. We don't hear about these suicides. They don't get reported on (out of precaution). They can't be explained by the limited research we have access to without people rushing to contest it, especially when the victims are heavily doped on prescription drugs and can't assert their rights.

I took it for granted none of the medical staff who'd been part of Ferid Ferkovic's story would take any responsibility for the health system's shortfalls—and I was right. From the very start, everything had been stacked against him; it had all contributed to the tragic death of someone so

young. The staff decided what was best, favour-
ing drugs over all other (less invasive, effective)
approaches. They systematically sabotaged our
efforts to bring Ferid back to himself under the
guise that they knew best. We'd slowly drawn
Ferid out of his shell. We'd gotten him to speak
with us again and even persuaded him that the
hospital was a place he could feel safe, even
though he'd been distrustful of it from the start.

I sent my son's case to the Collège des Méde-
cins du Québec, the province's professional order
of physicians, on September 25, 2015, naively
hoping they'd dig deeper than the Jewish General
had. But they rendered their verdict only after
reading my request filed with the review committee. The Collège studied Ferid's medical
file, the examiner's reply, then my request for a
review and concluded that the ER psychiatrist
had acted competently. Clearly the contradictions
between our two versions of events hadn't been
questioned.

There's not much point in continuing the
debate. This book is my response to what happened. I've spent long nights writing it, long days
putting my pain into words. And I've won in the
end. Ferid didn't die for nothing. He's still fighting, through me. And it's not over yet.

31. Support Through Dignity

The only real destination on a road to recovery is inner peace. We are all called to make the journey at some point in our lives. Whether it is in response to life's inevitable trials or just to stay alive. Ferid's final messages to me were clear, but I hadn't understood their true meaning at the time. The week before he died, he told me, "It's over now—I won't be a bother anymore." I'd thought at the time he was just worried about me. It'd been a relief to see him so calm. But clearly I missed a warning sign. I think we were all wounded at that point, each of us living in our own worlds. We were trying to survive. We were waiting... for what exactly? For nothing. For God in his mercy to deliver us.

It hadn't registered for me at the time that a great part of our misfortune wasn't fighting schizophrenia, it was fighting against the people who'd decided to "heal" Ferid as they thought fit. Sometimes I find myself sitting for hours trying to piece together the past in a way that makes sense. I've sought refuge by turning inward, and in writing. I have to finish what Ferid began and let the world know that it wasn't schizophrenia that pushed him to the edge. Far from it.

One afternoon my handsome son came up to me and said sweetly, "You know, Mom, up till now I thought a roof over your head and enough to eat was enough to be happy. But that's not living." I didn't know how to answer. The overwhelming powerlessness a parent feels at knowing they cannot change a situation—how do you put that into words? My memory is faulty. I don't remember what I said, or whether I tried to reassure him. But I know that sentence will be with me for the rest of my days.

In his vulnerability, my son became more open. He spent more time with us and expressed himself more often. In the kitchen, a place that holds so many sad memories, he once told me, "See how hunched over I am, Mom? I shouldn't look like this." He was starting to notice the debilitating effects of his illness, unaware—although I'm aware today—that it was not the only reason his health was failing; the toxic drugs he'd been prescribed were also at work.

When nature's complexity shifts how we see things, we are also forced to humility. Nature is an inscrutable mystery, despite the arrogance and impatience of some, who take it upon themselves to decide who deserves to live, to thrive, and who gets left behind. I learned this bitter truth through my time with an exceptional son who God gave me on Earth. We were unjustly told schizophrenia is incurable, and that was enough to extinguish our hope. "He'll never have a normal life, a job, or a family," the resident psychiatrist had once told my daughter. Those words could extinguish just about any life.

As of April 15, 2013, Ferid grew calmer. I can only remember those final quiet evenings—how perfect they were. I didn't see it coming. I'd placed my hope in Providence. At that point, I had only God left to trust in.

Acknowledgements

I would sincerely like to thank J.-Claude St-Onge for so carefully listening to me and for his invaluable help as I wrote this book. Thanks also to Kevin Boire of Action Autonomie for his unwavering support, to the French whistleblower Elena Pasca for her generosity, and to all the researchers and scientists whose work has nourished my reflection and provided the opportunity to share their so valuable knowledge with others. Warm thanks are also due to publisher Robin Philpot and his team at Baraka Books and Aleshia Jensen who translated this book. They took up the torch so that Ferid could "complete his mission," namely to build on people's inner strength and resilience so that hope will provide the unique route to be taken.

I dedicate this book to my father Hocine and my mother Hafsa.

Notes

Foreword

1. *Les fous crient au secours* is the story of a young insurance salesman who is committed against his will to a psychiatric ward in Saint-Jean-de-Dieu hospital in the early 1960s. The book was originally published by Éditions du jour in 1961 and republished by Écosociété in 2018. It received a great deal of attention in Quebec in the early days of the Quiet Revolution.

2. Psychiatric drugs must not be discontinued abruptly or without assistance, as is done in most drug-sponsored studies.

3. Jaakko Seikkula et al., "Five-Year Experience of First-Episode Nonaffective Psychosis in Open-Dialogue Approach: Treatment Principles, Follow-up Outcomes, and Two Case Studies," *Psychotherapy Research*, 16, no. 2, (March 2006): 214–228.

4. Michal M. Kłapciński and Joanna Rymaszewska, "Open Dialogue Approach – about the phenomenon of Scandinavian Psychiatry," Psychiatria Polska, 49, no. 6 (2015): 1179–1190.

5. Sera Davidow, "Hearing Voices in the USA," *Mad in America. Science, Psychiatry and Social Justice*, July 13, 2017, http://madinamerica.com/2017/07/hearing-voices-in-the-usa/.

6. Symptoms considered positive are hallucinations, delusion, and thought or behavioural problems. Negative symptoms include apathy, social withdrawal and affective flattening.

7. Joan-Ramon Laporte, "Un point brillant sur les neuroleptiques," *Bulletin d'informations de pharmacologie* (BIP31.fr), 24, no. 1, (April 2017): 10.

8. Jay Joseph, *The Gene Illusion: Genetic Research in Psychiatry and Psychology Under the Microscope*, (New York: Algora Publishing, 2004).

9. James P. Evans and Jonathan S. Berg, "The Value of Your Genome. Genome Sequencing: It's Not for Everyone," *The Scientist*, December 1, 2012.

10. Margaret C. Cutajar et al., "Schizophrenia and Other Psychotic Disorders in a Cohort of Sexually Abused Children," *Archives of General Psychiatry*, 67, No. 11 (November 2010).

11. Rebecca Pinto, Mark Asworth and Roger Jones, "Schizophrenia in black Caribbeans living in the UK: An exploration of underlying causes of the high incidence rate," *British Journal of General Practice*, 58, no. 551 (June 2008): 429–434.

4. Ferid: Before

1. Sadia Messaili, *La route de la dignité*, Saint-Jean-sur-Richelieu, Éditions JCL, 2005.

5. Ignorance

1. CQLR, chapter P-38.001, LégisQuébec, http://legisquebec. gouv.qc.ca/en/ShowDoc/cs/P-38.001.See also "Quels sont mes droits?" (What are my rights?) Action Autonomie, mental health rights advocacy group in Montreal, http://www.actionautonomie.qc.ca/category/droits-recours.

2. CQLR, chapter P-38.001.

8. First Hospitalization

1. 11-Neuroleptiques et autres antipsychotiques - PharmaEtudes https://www.yumpu.com/fr/document/view/41378864/11-neuroleptiques-et-autres-antipsychotiques-pharmaetudes

2. "Schizophrénie (psychose, troubles psychotiques)," *Salut Bonjour*, http://sante.canoe.ca/condition/getcondition/ schizophrenie.

3. Jean-Claude St-Onge, *Tous fous? L'influence de l'industrie pharmaceutique sur la psychiatrie*, Montréal, Écosociété, 2013, 223–224. (Are we all mad? The drug industry's influence on psychiatry).

4. Marie-Luce Quintal et al., *Je suis une personne, pas une maladie ! La maladie mentale, l'espoir d'un mieux-être*, (Longueuil: Performance Édition, 2013), 29.

5. Act respecting health and social services (section 3), LegisQuébec, http://legisquebec.gouv.qc.ca/en/ShowDoc/ cs/S-4.2.

6. Danielle Thibault, *Les contenus religieux du délire schizophrénique*, conference given to members of the AQPAMM, (October 26, 2011), 4.

9. Electroshock Treatment

1. Lawrence Stevens, "Psychiatry's Electroconvulsive Shock Treatment: A Crime Against Humanity," *Antipsychiatry*, updated in 1997, http://www.antipsychiatry.org/ect.htm.
2. Norman S. Sutherland, cited in Stevens, Ibid.
3. Peter R. Breggin, cited in Stevens, Ibid.
4. Karl H. Pribram, cited in Stevens, Ibid.
5. Sidney Sament, cited in Stevens, Ibid.
6. Agence d'évaluation des technologies et des modes d'intervention en santé, *L'utilisation des électrochocs au Québec*, report prepared by Reiner Banken for AÉTMIS, Sainte-Foy, Les publications du Québec, 2003, 9–10. (Translated citation).
7. Pare-Chocs, Comité pour l'abolition des électrochocs, *Info Choquée, Bulletin mensuel*, Vol. 3, No. 2 Avril 2010; https://www.actionautonomie.qc.ca/parechocs/pdf/bulletinvol3no2.pdf; accessed 13 March 2020.
8. St-Onge, *Tous fous?*, 125.

10. Reality on the Ground

1. "Jeunes et santé mentale" forum, *Pour un regard différent*, April 15, 2016, www.agidd.org/wp-content/uploads/2016/04/Resultats-consultation-Forum-Santementale-jeunes-1.pdf.

11. Home from the Hospital

1. Cited by Terence Young, Chair, Drug Safety Canada, speaking at the House Standing Committee on Health, March 6, 2008.
2. Terence Young, *Death by Prescription*, Toronto: Key Porter Books, 2009.
3. Young, *Death*, 137–138.
4. Tempra, *Ressources Santé*, https://www.ressourcessante.salutbonjour.ca/drug/getdrug/tempra.

12. Road to Recovery or Dead-End?

1. Luc Vigneault, "Les allers-retours d'un battant," Quintal et al., *Je suis une personne*, 38–39. (Translated citation).
2. Ibid., 42–44. (Translated citation).
3. Marie-Luce Quintal and Luc Vigneault, "Métissage d'expériences menant à une théorie de rétablissement," Quintal et al., *Je suis une personne*, 58. (Translated citation).
4. In her 1997 article "Breaking Down the Barriers," Dr. Leona Bachrach, citing John Talbott, M.D. and chair of the University

of Maryland School of Medicine, indicates the existence of more than 200 barriers to psychiatric care that workers in the homelessness support sector encounter daily. Cited by Marie-Carmen Plante, "Les maux de la psychiatrie face à l'itinérance," Roy and Hurtubise (eds.), *L'itinérance en questions* (Québec: Presses de l'université du Québec, 2007). 217–232.

5. Ibid., 217–232.

6. Comorbidity and polymorbidity are the coexistence of two or more pathologies in the same patient, which can result from an initial illness.

7. Plante, "Les maux," 243–258. (Translated citation).

8. Ibid, 220–21. (Translated citation).

13. Drug-Free Treatment

1. Patricia E. Deegan, "Recovery as a Self-Directed Process of Healing and Transformation," *Occupational Therapy in Mental Health* 17 (2008): 5–21. doi: 10.1300/J004v17n03_02

2. Patricia E. Deegan, "The Lived Experience of Rehabilitation," *Psychosocial Rehabilitation Journal* 11 (1988): 14–15.

3. Robert Whitaker, "The Door to a Revolution in Psychiatry Cracks Open: Norway's Health Ministry Orders Medication-Free Treatment," *Mad in America*, March 25, 2017, www.madinamerica. com/2017/03/the-door-to-a-revolution-in-psychiatry-cracks-open.

4. Ibid.

5. *Open Dialogue: An Alternative, Finnish Approach to Healing Psychosis*, directed by Daniel Mackler, 2011, https://www.youtube.com/watch?v=HDVhZHJagfQ.

6. *Open Dialogue: An International Community* (website), accessed February 14, 2020, http://open-dialogue.net/.

7. Mackler, *Open Dialogue*.

8. Ibid.

14. Three Years of Remission

1. St-Onge, *Tous fous?*, 42.

2. Young, *Death by Prescription*.

15. Zyprexa

1. J.-Claude St-Onge, *L'envers de la pilule. Les dessous de l'industrie pharmaceutique* (Montréal: Écosociété, 2008), 269. (Translated citation).

2. Taken from *Prescrire*, "Effets indésirables métaboliques de l'olanzapine: procès en cascade aux États-Unis," *Prescrire* 28 (15 March 2008), 224-226.

3. Elena Pasca, "Procès Zyprexa : charge virulente du juge contre les autorités sanitaires qui ont laissé faire Eli Lilly," *Pharmacritique, 20minutes* (blog), July 23, 2008, http://pharmacritique.20minutes-blogs.fr/archive/2008/07/23/debut-du-proces-zyprexa-le-juge-denonce-la-faillitedes-auto.html.

4. Ibid.

5. Oral Statement by the Court at Class Cert. *In re Zyprexa Prods. Liab. Litig.*, Hr'g, *83 (E.D.N.Y.) July 17, 2008, Docket No. 05-CV-411

6. J.-Claude St-Onge, *Les dérives de l'industrie de la santé: Petit abécédaire* (Montréal, Écosociété, 2006), 201; Jeffrey A. Lieberman et al., "Effectiveness of Antipsychotic Drugs in Patients with Chronic Schizophrenia," *New England Journal of Medicine* 353 (September 22, 2005), 1209. DOI: 10.1056/NEJMoa051688

7. David Healy, "Randomized Controlled Trials: Evidence Biased Psychiatry," *Alliance for Human Research Protection* online, October 26, 2006, www.ahrp.org/COI/healy0802.php.

8. St-Onge, *Les dérives*, 202–203. (Translated citation).

9. The information in this paragraph is taken from St-Onge, *Tous fous?*, 124–125.

10. Robert Whitaker, "Harrow + Wunderink + Open Dialogue = An Evidence-based Mandate for A New Standard of Care," *Mad in America*, July 17, 2013, https://www.madinamerica.com/2013/07/harrow-wunkerlink-open-dialogue-an-evidence-based-mandate-for-a-new-standard-of-care/

11. For more information on Open Dialogue, see Chapter 13.

12. For these studies see: https://jamanetwork.com/journals/jamapsychiatry/fullarticle/1707650 and https://www.ncbi.nlm.nih.gov/pubmed/17502806

13. Benzodiazepines are a class of psychoactive drugs used for anxiety disorders and sleep problems.

14. Joan-Ramon Laporte, "Un point brillant sur les neuroleptiques," BIP31.fr (April 2017), 10, www.bip31.fr/bip/BIP31.fr%20 2017,%2024,%20(1),%201-15.pdf. (Translated citation).

15. Peter C. Gøtzsche, *Deadly Medicines and Organised Crime* (London, Radcliffe, 2013), 199.

16. Pharmed Out, "Zyprexa drug rep," YouTube video, https://www.youtube.com/watch?time_continue=1&v=nj0LZZzrcrs&feature=emb_logo

16. Schizophrenia

1. Allen Frances, *Saving Normal: An Insider's Revolt against Out-of-Control Psychiatric Diagnosis, DSM-5, Big Pharma, and the Medicalization of Ordinary Life* (New York: William Morrow, an imprint of HarperCollins Publishers, 2013), 21.
2. Thomas S. Szasz, *Schizophrenia: The Sacred Symbol of Psychiatry*, (NYC: Basic Books, 1976).
3. World Health Organization, "Schizophrenia," https://who.int/news-room/fact-sheets/detail/schizophrenia.
4. Public Heath Agency of Canada, "Chapter 3: Schizophrenia," *Report on Mental Illnesses in Canada,* October 2002, 49.
5. This is obviously one of many factors that leads young people with schizophrenia to commit suicide. Other factors including the stigma attached to the illness, limited or non-existant access to employement, a lack of alternative resources, isolation, drug side effects, inadequate care in hospital emergency rooms during episodes, etc.
6. Public Health Agency, *Report on Mental Illnesses*, 52–53.
7. Cited in Wayne Ramsay (a.k.a Lawrence Stevens), "Schizophrenia: A Nonexistent Disease," http://wayneramsay.com/schizophrenia.htm.
8. Ramsay, "Schizophrenia."
9. Allen J. Frances, "No Child Left Undiagnosed: The Latest Ploy to Make Childhood a Disease," *Psychology Today*, April 12, 2014, https://psychologytoday.com/blog/saving-normal/201404/no-child-left-undiagnosed.
10. J.-Claude St-Onge, *TDAH? Pour en finir avec le dopage des enfants*, (Montreal: Écosociété, 2015), 25.
11. For further reading: *Tous hyperactifs ?* by Patrick Landman (Paris: Albin Michel, 2015) and *TDAH ?* by St-Onge.

18. Relapse

1. Abla Farhoud, *Le fou d'Omar* (Montreal: VLB, 2005), 88–89. (Translated citation).

19. Ferid, aka Jesus Christ: A Second Psychotic Episode

1. William Anthony, "Recovery from Mental Illness: The Guiding Vision of the Mental Health Service System in the 1990s," *Psychological Rehabilitation Journal*, 16, no. 4 (April 1993): 11. Cited in Quintal et al., *Je suis une personne*, 61.

2. Hélène Provencher, "L'expérience du rétablissement : perspectives théoriques." *Santé mentale au Québec*, 27, no. 1 (spring 2002), 35–64. Cited in Quintal et al., *Je suis une personne*. (Translated Citation).

20. Court Authorization for Treatment

1. *Civil Code of Québec*, Article 10, LegisQuébec, http://legisque-bec.gouv.qc.ca/en/showdoc/cs/CCQ-1991.

2. In Quebec the legal age of consent is 14. That said, I do not know many children that age who have the necessary faculties of reason to give their free and enlightened consent.

3. Remember that Ferid had been told he would lose his bed if he didn't take his medication.

4. Association des groupes d'intervention en défense des droits en santé mentale du Québec, "L'autorisation judiciaire de soins : le trou noir de la psychiatrie. Étude et analyse de 150 jugements, réflexions sur la pratique et recommandations de l'AGIDD-SMQ." Montreal, May 2014. (Court mandated care: psychiatry's black hole. Study and analysis of 150 judgments, reflections on practice and the AGIDD-SMQ's recommendations.)

5. Ibid., 5. (Translated citation).

6. Ibid., 5, 29–30. (Translated citation).

21. Meeting the Social Worker, or Autoposy of an Act of Sabotage

1. Marie-Laurence Poirel, "Entretien avec Marie-Luce Quintal, psychiatre, Centre de traitement et de réadaptation de Nemours (CTR) de Québec," *Santé mentale au Québec* 36, no. 1 (spring 2011): 99–113. (Translated citation).

2. Suzanne Lamarre, *Le suicide, l'affaire de tous. Vers une nouvelle approche*, (Montreal: Éditions de l'Homme, 2014), 41–42.

3. Ibid, 42. (Translated citation).

4. Information in this paragraph taken from: FFAPAMM, "Votre collègue de travail a une maladie mentale... Son comportement vous inquiète ?," *Réseau Avant de craquer*, communiqué, October 5, 2009.

22. Other Options

1. André Paradis, "En mémoire des années 70," in Yves Lecomte (Ed.), *20 ans de santé mentale au Québec. Regards critiques des acteurs et des collaborateurs*, special edition of *Santé mentale et société*, 1996, 29. (Translated citation).
2. In a paternalistic relationship, medical professionals hold a great deal of power over the patient's life, since they handle the whole of their needs from creating treatment plans to choosing where the person will live, including their professional and personal activities.
3. "Managerial Communication Techniques: Defining Active Listening – Carl Rogers," http://www.HR4free.com/en.
4. Quintal et al., *Je suis une personne*, 81. (Translated citation).

25. April 15, 2013

1. Brian Mishara and Michel Tousignant, *Comprendre le suicide*, (Montreal: Presses de l'Université de Montréal, 2004) 60.
2. American Psychiatric Association, *Diagnostic and Statistical Manual of Mental Disorders (DSM-5®)*, 2013.

26. Life After Ferid

1. Peter C. Gøtzsche, *Deadly Medicines and Organised Crime: How Big Pharma Has Corrupted Healthcare*, Radcliffe Publishing, 2013.
2. *BMJ 2015; 351 doi: https://doi.org/10.1136/bmj.h4320*
3. *The Guardian*, August 27, 2004.
4. "L'antidépresseur paroxétine des laboratoires Glaxo inefficace et risqué pour les adolescents. Une étude publiée dans le British Medical Journal dénonce les résultats d'une précédente étude financée par le laboratoire," *Le Monde* avec AFP, September 19, 2015.
5. Gøtzsche, *Deadly Medicines*, 220.
6. Ibid, 220–1.
7. Gøtzsche, *Deadly Medicines*, 259.
8. Olivier Pighetti, *Morts sur ordonnance* (Prescription death), Piments Pourpres Productions, 2014, 52 minutes. Documentary available on YouTube.
9. Peter R. Breggin, MD – Antidepressants & Suicide – Congressional Testimony," February 12, 2011, http://youtube.com/watch?v=SBJfZtB_3cc.

10. Peter R. Breggin, *Medication Madness: The Role of Psychiatric Drugs in Cases of Violence, Suicide and Crime*, (New York: St. Martin's Griffin, 2009).

27. Fighting Fatalism
1. Frances, *Saving Normal*, 105.
2. Ibid, 96.
3. See, https://www.baumhedlundlaw.com/bristol-myers-abilify-settlement-19-billion/

28. Filing a Complaint: The Long Wait
1. Annual Report of the Québec Ombudsman for fiscal year 2014-2015, presented at the National Assembly, September 2015, https://protecteurducitoyen.qc.ca/sites/default/files/pdf/rapports_annuels/annual-report-protecteur-2014-2015.pdf.
2. Ministère de la Santé et des Services sociaux du Québec, *Modèle de protocole de mise sous garde en établissement de santé et de services sociaux des personnes dangereuses pour elles-mêmes ou pour autrui en raison de leur état mental* (Protocol for confinement of persons whose mental state presents a danger to themselves or to others), December 19, 2018, http://publications.msss.gouv.qc.ca/msss/document-002234.
3. Daniel Mackler, *Take These Broken Wings*, 115 minutes, 2008. The English version of this documentary has been viewed over 235 thousand times on YouTube (2020), which is quite an impressive number given the subject matter.
4. Joanne Greenberg is the author of 16 novels, including *I Never Promised You a Rose Garden* (New York: Holt, Rinehart and Winston, 1964). Screen adaptation in 1977 by Anthony Page.

29. Duty to Rescue
1. The examiner's reply is dated April 7, 2016. It was posted on April 21st and I received it the 24th. By law my complaint should have been dealt with in 45 days.
2. I would later discover that sending suffering, suicidal and psychiatrically diagnosed people home was common practice in the emergency room! It seems that they even send people home who have been escorted there by police.

ALSO FROM BARAKA BOOKS

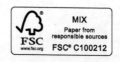

Printed by Imprimerie Gauvin
Gatineau, Québec